P9-CNI-000

Fight
Alzheimer's
with Vitamins and
Antioxidants

"Fight Alzheimer's with Vitamins and Antioxidants by Kedar Prasad, Ph.D., contains clinically and scientifically valid information presented in an easy-to-follow format that informs the reader about the value of vitamins, antioxidants, and micronutrients in preventing and/or slowing the symptoms of Alzheimer's disease. It captures up-to-date scientific information on the pathology of Alzheimer's disease and the state of its therapy and presents a straightforward argument on the values of vitamins and antioxidants.

"The tables that show dietary reference intakes (DRI) are a great feature. The information allows the text to serve as a source of reference, supplying data that readers can use to make their own judgments about dosages of vitamins and antioxidants."

CLIVEL G. CHARLTON, PH.D., DIRECTOR FOR THE
CENTER FOR MOLECULAR AND BEHAVIORAL NEUROSCIENCE
COLLEGE OF MEDICINE AT MEHARRY MEDICAL COLLEGE

"Fight Alzheimer's with Vitamins and Antioxidants offers a simple and inexpensive means to delay the onset and progression of the disease. This safe, straightforward approach involves readily accessible vitamins and other micronutrients. Prasad's book is full of valid and excellent suggestions on how to interfere with the evolution of Alzheimer's. I strongly recommend this book."

STEPHEN C. BONDY, PH.D., PROFESSOR,
DEPARTMENT OF MEDICINE, UNIVERSITY OF CALIFORNIA

Fight
Alzheimer's
with **Vitamins** and
Antioxidants

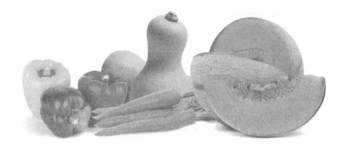

Kedar N. Prasad, Ph.D.

Healing Arts Press
Rochester, Vermont • Toronto, Canada

Healing Arts Press
One Park Street
Rochester, Vermont 05767
www.HealingArtsPress.com

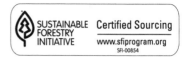

Text stock is SFI certified

Healing Arts Press is a division of Inner Traditions International

Copyright © 2015 by Kedar N. Prasad, Ph.D.

Note to the reader: This book is intended as an informational guide. The remedies, approaches, and techniques described herein are meant to supplement, and not to be a substitute for, professional medical care or treatment. They should not be used to treat a serious ailment without prior consultation with a qualified health care professional.

Library of Congress Cataloging-in-Publication Data
Prasad, Kedar N.
  Fight Alzheimer's with vitamins and antioxidants / Kedar N. Prasad, Ph.D.
      pages cm
    Summary: "The most complete and up-to-date resource on the powerful benefits of nutritional supplements for the treatment and prevention of Alzheimer's disease" — Provided by publisher.
  Includes bibliographical references and index.
  ISBN 978-1-62055-317-6 (paperback) — ISBN 978-1-62055-318-3 (e-book)
  1. Alzheimer's disease—Treatment. 2. Vitamin therapy. 3. Antioxidants—Therapeutic use. I. Title.
  RC523.P735 2015
  616.8'31—dc23

                                                                    2014042437

Printed and bound in the United States by Lake Book Manufacturing, Inc.
The text stock is SFI certified. The Sustainable Forestry Initiative® program promotes sustainable forest management.

10 9 8 7 6 5 4 3 2 1

Text design and layout by Virginia Scott Bowman
This book was typeset in Garamond Premier Pro and Frutiger with Avant Garde and Helvetica Neue used as the display typeface

To send correspondence to the author of this book, mail a first-class letter to the author c/o Inner Traditions • Bear & Company, One Park Street, Rochester, VT 05767, and we will forward the communication, or contact the author directly at **kprasad@mypmcinside.com.**

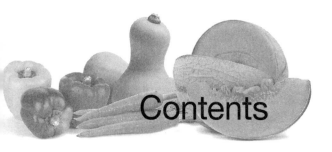

Contents

ACKNOWLEDGMENTS

I would like to thank my family for their support and encouragement. I also am very thankful to Anne Dillon and Chanc VanWinkle Orzell for their superb editing of this book.

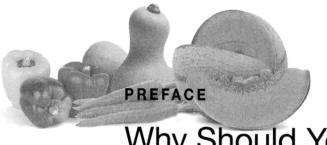

Why Should You Read This Book?

Alzheimer's disease, a progressive disorder that attacks the neurons in the brain, accounts for 60 to 80 percent of all dementia cases. Although it typically affects older individuals, it also can affect younger people carrying mutated genes; indeed up to 5 percent of individuals afflicted with Alzheimer's disease have what is known as "early onset Alzheimer's," which can present with symptomatology when individuals are in their 40s or 50s. This is due to a familial Alzheimer's in which mutations in certain genes cause the onset of this disease earlier. Symptoms of Alzheimer's disease may include memory loss, a decrease in problem-solving abilities, difficulty completing ordinary chores and tasks, confusion, depression, spatial disorientation, difficulty speaking or writing, losing things, poor judgment, social withdrawal, and mood changes.

Alzheimer's disease remains a major medical concern in the United States, given that it strikes primarily older people (age sixty-five and over). This demographic is expected to increase from about 40.2 million in 2010 to about 89 million by the year 2050 (U.S. Census Bureau, 2010). Consequently, this disease will create huge health problems and be a burden on society in terms of the cost of its management.

At present, there is no adequate strategy for the prevention of Alzheimer's disease, and its treatment options remain unsatisfactory. In this book I propose a unified hypothesis that increased oxidative stress and chronic inflammation are primarily responsible for the initiation and progression of this disease. Therefore, mitigating oxidative stress and chronic inflammation appears to be a logical solution to reduce the disease's development and progression. The proposed strategy, in combination with standard therapy, may improve management outcomes more than just utilizing standard therapy alone.

In order to reduce oxidative stress and chronic inflammation, it's essential to increase the body's levels of all antioxidant enzymes and all standard dietary and endogenous antioxidants.* This goal cannot be achieved by the use of the one or two antioxidants that have been used in clinical studies for the prevention or treatment of in some neurodegenerative diseases in humans. Therefore, I have proposed that a preparation of micronutrients containing *multiple* dietary and endogenous antioxidants, B vitamins with high doses of vitamin B$_3$ (nicotinamide), vitamin D, selenium, and certain polyphenolic compounds (curcumin and resveratrol) should be employed in clinical studies for reducing the risk of development and progression of Alzheimer's disease. These micronutrients are capable of increasing the levels of all antioxidant enzymes by activating a nuclear transcriptional factor-2/antioxidant response element (Nrf2/ARE) pathway, as well as by enhancing the levels of standard dietary and endogenous antioxidants.

Most neurologists believe that antioxidants and vitamins have no significant role to play in the prevention or the improved management of Alzheimer's disease. These beliefs are primarily based on a few clinical studies in which supplementation with a single antioxidant, such as vitamin E, produced modest beneficial effects or no effect. However, the brains of patients with a neurodegenerative disease such as Alzheimer's may be a characterized by a high oxidative environment. Therefore,

---

*Endogenous antioxidants are antioxidants that are made by the body.

the administration of a single antioxidant should *not be expected* to produce any significant beneficial effect. This is because an individual antioxidant in the presence of a highly oxidative environment may be oxidized to act as a pro-oxidant rather than an antioxidant. Coupled with this is the fact that levels of the oxidized form of the antioxidant may increase after the prolonged consumption of the single antioxidant. This increase can damage brain cells. In addition, a single antioxidant can't enhance the levels of antioxidant enzymes as well as the levels of dietary and endogenous antioxidants.

In peer-reviewed journals I have published several reviews that challenge the current trend of using a single antioxidant for the prevention and/or management of neurodegenerative diseases in high-risk populations. These articles have failed to have any significant impact on the design of clinical trials, however, and the inconsistent results of the effects of a single antioxidant continue to be published. And although some books on neurodegenerative diseases and their causes and symptoms are available, none of them have critically analyzed the published data on the effects of antioxidants on neurodegenerative diseases. Nor have they questioned whether the experimental designs of the study on which the conclusions were based were scientifically valid; whether the results obtained from the use of a single antioxidant in a high-risk population may be extrapolated to the effect of the same antioxidant in a multiple antioxidant preparation for the same population; or whether the results of studies obtained on high-risk populations can be extrapolated to normal populations.

The growing controversies regarding the value of multiple micronutrients in the prevention and improved management of neurodegenerative diseases need to be addressed, and new solutions need to be proposed. This book articulates the reasons for the controversies mentioned above and proposes evidence and scientifically based, rational solutions for the prevention and improved management of Alzheimer's disease.

To set us on the right track, we must first begin with clinical studies that utilize a preparation of various micronutrients, not just one or two. The validity of this expanded approach is supported by two recent clinical studies pertaining to other diseases. In contrast to previous studies in which supplementation with beta-carotene alone increased the risk of lung cancer among heavy tobacco smokers, two clinical studies utilizing a preparation of multiple antioxidants revealed a reduced incidence of cancer by 10 percent and an improved clinical outcome in patients with HIV/AIDS. These studies were published in the *Journal of the American Medical Association* (JAMA), a very prestigious medical journal.

A comprehensive preparation of micronutrients containing multiple dietary and endogenous antioxidants, B vitamins, vitamin D, selenium, and certain polyphenolic compounds (curcumin and resveratrol) for the prevention and/or improved management of a neurodegenerative disease such as Alzheimer's, in conjunction with standard therapy, has never been proposed.

I have done so in this book.

Herein I discuss oxidative stress and inflammation as well as the properties and function of antioxidants and certain phenolic compounds; the structure and function of the normal human brain; and the incidence, cost, and cause of Alzheimer's disease. In so doing, in Table 7.1, I present a formulation of micronutrients containing multiple dietary and endogenous antioxidants and B vitamins, vitamin D, selenium, and certain polyphenolic compounds (curcumin and resveratrol) that may be helpful in the prevention and management of Alzheimer's. These substances have been used by consumers for decades without reported toxicity.

Also in the book, in the appendix, are tables that advise the reader as to recommended dosages of micronutrients for everyday health and well-being. I hope the information contained herein will serve as a guide to those who are interested in using micronutrients to reduce the risk of developing Alzheimer's disease and/or retard its progression.

Laboratory data suggests that even the genetic basis of neurological diseases can be prevented or delayed by micronutrient supplements.

Primary care physicians and practicing neurologists interested in complementary medicine may discover that my findings are useful in recommending micronutrient supplements for their patients. Consumers who are taking daily supplements will find the information provided in this book encouraging. Those who are not taking supplements or are uncertain as to their potential benefits may find evidence to help them make a decision about whether or not to take micronutrient supplements daily, in consultation with their doctors.

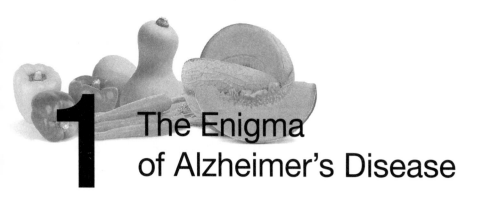

1
The Enigma
of Alzheimer's Disease

Alzheimer's disease is a form of neurodegenerative disease characterized by the progressive loss of nerve cells from the cortex region of the brain. It is the main causative agent of memory loss (dementia), and it progresses slowly.* Individuals who are sixty-five years of age or older are at risk of developing Alzheimer's disease; in the United States it is the sixth leading cause of death among people of this demographic. In 90 percent of cases the disease is acquired; only in 5 to 10 percent of cases is it inherited.

When Alzheimer's strikes the damaged neurons of the brain render memory less reliable. Cognitive thinking, language skills, and one's judgment are negatively impacted, and behavioral changes in the individual suffering from the disease are apt to be noted. Those with the disease tend to live, on average, for another eight years after their symptoms have become apparent, although this range can be anywhere from four years to twenty years, depending on other factors.

A diagnosis of Alzheimer's disease is made by postmortem analysis of the brains of patients with dementia. A chief marker of Alzheimer's disease is what is known as a neurofibrillary tangle (NFT), which is a

---

*Other types of dementia include vascular dementia, mixed dementia, dementia with Lewy bodies, Parkinson's disease with dementia, frontotemporal dementia, and alcoholic dementia. Like Alzheimer's disease, most types of dementia are acquired, with only a small percentage of them being due to a family history (familial type).

conglomeration of proteins known as hyperphosphorylated tau protein and apolipoprotein E. Neurofibrillary tangles, found inside the nerve cells of the cortex region of the brain, are insoluble and are difficult to degrade by proteolytic enzymes. Senile (neuritic) plaques located outside of the nerve cells in the brain containing several proteins are also considered hallmarks of Alzheimer's disease (Yankner and Mesulam 1991; Selkoe 1994; Kudo et al. 1994). Neuritic plaques are focal and spherical, and their size ranges from 20 to 200 microns in diameter. Activated microglia and astrocytes (markers of chronic inflammation) are present at the periphery of the plaques.

When one has Alzheimer's disease the synaptic connections between nerve cells are often lost. Interestingly, a study has shown that Lewy bodies—bundles of proteins that manifest inside nerve cells and are characteristic of Parkinson's disease—are also present in the brains of approximately 60 percent of Alzheimer's cases (Hamilton 2000).

The mechanisms of the formation and dissolution of neurofibrillary tangles and plaques are under extensive investigation so that new drugs to improve treatment outcomes may be developed. Currently, there is no known cure for this puzzling disease. However, it's my belief that increased oxidative stress and chronic inflammation are primarily responsible for its initiation and progression; therefore, attenuation of these biochemical defects may reduce the risk of development and progression of this disease and, in combination with standard therapy, improve the clinical outcomes.

This chapter discusses briefly the history, prevalence/incidence, and cost of Alzheimer's disease. We then move on to a general discussion of oxidative stress and chronic inflammation and examine how these processes affect the body so that we may better understand their role. In the next chapter we'll explore the human brain, before returning, in chapter 3, to a deeper discussion of oxidative stress and inflammation as they pertain to the manifestation of Alzheimer's disease.

HISTORY, PREVALENCE/INCIDENCE, AND COST TO SOCIETY

History

Progressive memory loss (forgetfulness) has been known for centuries. Claudius Galen, a Roman physician who lived during the second century, described the age-related symptoms of absentmindedness. In the fourteenth century in England, a verbal test was utilized to evaluate one's level of memory loss. In 1906 Dr. Alois Alzheimer, a German psychologist, cared for a fifty-one-year-old female who was suffering from severe memory loss associated with confusion. After her death he performed an autopsy on her brain and noted the presence of dense deposits (senile plaques*) outside of its nerve cells, as well as twisted bands of fibers (neurofibrillary tangles) inside the nerve cells.

Subsequently, Dr. Alzheimer's colleague, Dr. Emil Kraepelin, coined the term "Alzheimer's disease." He was so impressed with Alzheimer's research that he appointed him head of pathology at the Psychiatric Institute in Munich, Germany (now the Max Planck Institute). In 1960 neuroscientists discovered a link between memory loss and the presence of senile plaques and neurofibrillary tangles. Later, several biochemical and genetic defects that play a central role in the initiation and progression of Alzheimer's disease were identified.

Prevalence/Incidence

The term "prevalence" in a medical context is a measurement of how many cases of a disease exist in the population at a given time frame, whereas "incidence" refers to the number of cases of a disease that *develop* every year. It's estimated that in the United States, approximately 200,000 people under the age of sixty-five have Alzheimer's disease (Alzheimer's Disease Facts and Figures, Alzheimer's Association

---

*Extracellular senile plaque in the brain contains several proteins, including beta-amyloid, APOE, alpha-synuclein, and presenilins, and serves as a constant source of chronic inflammation in Alzheimer's patients.

2013). In 2014 5.2 million people age sixty-five or older suffer from it as well (3.2 million women and 1.8 million men). This represents 11 percent of people age sixty-five or over. By 2050 it is estimated that about 16 million Americans may suffer from this disease, if no breakthrough in prevention occurs. The incidence of Alzheimer's and other types of dementia (memory loss) doubles every five years for those individuals in this group (age sixty-five or older).

About 16 percent of women age seventy-one or older have Alzheimer's disease or another form of dementia, compared with only 11 percent of men in the same age group. This suggests that women are more prone to develop Alzheimer's than men. Additionally, approximately 30 percent of the U.S. population age eighty-five and older have symptoms of this disease (Alzheimer's Organization 2014).

INCIDENCE OF ALZHEIMER'S DISEASE*

Age (years)	New cases/year/1,000 people
65–74	53
75–84	173
85 or older	231

*From Alzheimer's Disease Facts and Figures, Alzheimer's Association 2013

According to a 2010 U.S. Census Bureau report, by 2030 one individual in five will be over the age of sixty-five, and in 2050 the number of Americans age sixty-five and older is projected to be 88.5 million. Currently, there is no cure for Alzheimer's. Consequently, in excess of half a million seniors die each year from this disease. Thus, it remains a major medical concern now as well as for future generations (U.S. Census Bureau, U.S. Department of Commerce 2010).

Cost to Society

At this time Alzheimer's disease is the most expensive disease in the United States. According to the U.S. Census Bureau, costs of the disease to society, in 2014, were projected to be an estimated $214 billion annually (please see the breakout below). By 2050 Alzheimer's is expected to cost $1.2 trillion per year (Alzheimer's Disease Facts and Figures, Alzheimer's Association 2013).

COST OF HEALTH AND LONG-TERM CARE SERVICES PER YEAR

Medicare	$113 billion
Medicaid	$37 billion
Out-of-pocket costs	$36 billion
Other sources: (HMOs, private insurance, managed care organizations, and uncompensated care)	$28 billion
Total	**$214 billion**

Despite extensive research and the publication of thousands of research studies on the causes of Alzheimer's, it has not been possible to reduce the incidence or the rate of progression of this disease. However, these studies have identified some biochemical and genetic defects that contribute to the death of nerve cells in the brain of Alzheimer's patients. Among these defects increased oxidative-stress-induced damage is one of the earliest biochemical markers indicating a degeneration of the brain's nerve cells (Prasad and Bondy, 2014).

Oxidative stress occurs when free radicals overwhelm the protective antioxidant systems of the body. These systems are composed of antioxidant enzymes and dietary and endogenous antioxidant chemicals. Increased oxidative stress due to production of excessive amounts of free radicals derived from oxygen and nitrogen play a pivotal role in the development and progression of damage in neurodegenerative diseases such as Alzheimer's disease and Parkinson's disease. Other biochemical and genetic defects occur subsequent to increased oxidative stress. Together these combined factors participate in an escalating cascade to progress the development of Alzheimer's in any given individual. Therefore, a basic understanding of oxidative stress and these other defects is essential for developing preventive and improved management strategies for Alzheimer's disease.

Before delving into that, however, let's look at the human immune system and the very important part it plays.

THE HUMAN IMMUNE SYSTEM

The immune system is a network of cells, tissues, and organs that work together in a highly coordinated manner to defend the body against foreign invading pathogenic (harmful) organisms and antigenic molecules and particles. As such, the immune system is essential for our survival. It is, however, also a double-edged sword. On the one hand it acts in the aforementioned defensive capacity. On the other hand it has the ability to produce chemicals that are toxic to the tissues. These chemicals include reactive oxygen species (ROS), which are free radicals derived from oxygen. Other chemicals that may be toxic to the tissues are pro-inflammatory cytokines, complement proteins, adhesion molecules, and prostaglandins, all of which may increase the risk of chronic diseases, including neurodegenerative diseases.

The organs of the immune system are located throughout the body and include lymphoid organs, which contain lymphocytes. Bone marrow is another important constituent of the body's immune system. It contains all of the body's blood cells, including lymphocytes. Thymus-derived lymphocytes are referred to as T-lymphocytes (T-cells). In the blood T-cells represent about 60 to 70 percent of peripheral lymphocytes.

Lymphocytes derived from bone marrow are referred to as B-lymphocytes (B-cells). They constitute about 10 to 20 percent of peripheral lymphocytes in the blood. B-cells mature to plasma cells, which secrete specific antibodies in response to a particular antigen.

Another type of cell that is germane to our discussion here is the neutrophil, which is formed from stem cells in the bone marrow. Likewise, macrophages are derived from monocytes of bone marrow and are part of the mononuclear phagocyte system. Macrophages exhibit phagocytic activity, which is essential for removing harmful organisms from the body. Macrophages and neutrophils are the most active in phagocytosis, following infection with pathogenic microorganisms.

Other types of cells play important roles, too. Natural killer (NK) cells represent about 10 to 15 percent of the peripheral blood lymphocytes but lack T-cell receptors. Like macrophages, they identify and kill harmful microorganisms by phagocytosis. Natural killer cells engulf pathogens that are trapped in an intracellular vesicle called a phagosome, which fuses with lysosomes to form phagolysosomes. The harmful organisms are killed by proteolytic enzymes (enzymes that can digest) of the lysosomes, aided by bursts of reactive oxygen species released by the phagocytes. Natural killer cells can kill tumor cells or cells infected with viruses.

A specialized form of cells with numerous fine dendritic cytoplasmic processes, called dendritic cells, do not exhibit phagocytic activity. Nevertheless, they play an important role in presenting antigen to T-cells.

Now that we understand a bit more about the components of a healthy immune system, let's take a look at the two basic modalities of immunity: innate immunity and adaptive immunity.

Innate Immunity

The innate immune defense is nonspecific and is the dominant system of host defense (Litman, Cannon, and Dishaw 2005). The innate immune system responds to infection by inducing inflammation, releasing complement proteins, and recruiting leukocytes. Leukocytes include the phagocytes (primarily macrophages and neutrophils), dendritic cells, mast cells, eosinophils, basophils, and natural killer cells (some of which are discussed above). The response of the innate immune system to infection is activated when microorganisms are identified by their pattern of recognition receptors or when damaged cells send signals to the immune system in order that a defensive response is generated

(Medzhitov 2007; Matzinger 2002). The innate immune responses do not confer long-lasting immunity against pathogenic organisms.

Adaptive Immunity

Adaptive immunity operates differently in that the lymphocytes (T-cells and B-cells) are responsible for the adaptive immune response. In adaptive immunity the presence of endogenous antigens can initiate an immune response that damages the body's own tissue, as in the case of rheumatoid arthritis, for instance. The immune system, once exposed to an antigen that it then successfully removes, stores the recognition factor of this antigen in its memory. Thus, during the lifetime of an individual, the immune system stores recognition factors of millions of different antigens, thereby protecting the body from these antigens all the time. This process of exposure to an antigen and then successfully removing it is generally referred to as "acquired immunity"—a form of adaptive immunity. As such, acquired immunity is the basis of vaccination.

The adaptive response to an antigen is strong. Its function is to store and recall immunologic memory in order to recognize and eliminate threatening antigens on a continual basis.

Both T-cells and B-cells carry receptors that recognize specific targets. T-cells can recognize only membrane-bound antigens, however. The cell surface major histocompatibility complex (MHC) molecules bind peptide fragments of foreign proteins for presentation to appropriate antigen-specific T-cells. There are two major subtypes of T-cells: the killer T-cells and the helper T-cells. The killer T-cells can recognize antigens bound to Class I MHC molecules, whereas the helper cells recognize antigens bound to Class II MHC molecules. A minor subtype of T-cells are the $\gamma\delta$ T-cells, which recognize intact antigens that are not bound to MHC receptors.

In contrast to the T-cell the surface of the B-cell has an antibody molecule for a specific antigen. The antibody molecules recognize whole harmful organisms and do not need any antigen-presenting mechanisms for their action. Each lineage of B-cell expresses a different antibody. A B-cell first identifies pathogens (harmful microorganisms) when an antibody on its surface binds to a specific foreign antigen. This antibody/antigen complex is engulfed by the B-cell, where it is converted into peptides by proteolytic enzymes. On their surface the B-cells then display antigenic peptides and Class II MHC molecules that attract matching T-helper cells, which release lymphokines and activate B-cells.

The activated B-cells proliferate and differentiate to plasma cells that secrete millions of copies of the antibody that recognize this antigen. These antibodies circulate in the blood and the lymph and bind to pathogens expressing this particular antigen. These antibody/antigen-bound pathogens are destroyed by complement protein activation or by phagocytes. Antibodies can also neutralize bacterial toxins by directly binding to them. They kill bacteria and viruses by interfering with their receptors, which are used to infect cells.

DAMAGING PROCESSES AND AGENTS IN THE BODY

Now that we understand a little something about the human immune system, let's look at agents and processes that damage the body. Oxidative stress is at the top of the list, and because of this we'll look at it first. In this we will briefly discuss how oxidative stress is precipitated by free radicals and the types and sources of those free radicals. We will also look at the process of inflammation. These issues are huge and complex, but I've attempted to describe them in simple and general terms here.

Oxidative Stress

Oxidative stress is a process that transpires when our protective antioxidant systems are eclipsed by an excessive production of free radicals derived from oxygen. Similarly, nitrosylative stress occurs when the generation of reactive nitrogen species exceeds the ability of the body's antioxidant defense system to neutralize them. Ongoing increases in oxidative and nitrosylative stress have been implicated in the initiation and progression of most chronic diseases* in humans wherein our protective antioxidant system has been breached and overwhelmed.

Let's backtrack through history for a moment to shed some light on the origins of the protective antioxidant system in the human body. At the dawn of time Earth's atmosphere had no oxygen. Tiny anaerobic organisms, which can live without oxygen, were thriving. About 2.5 billion years ago blue-green algae in the ocean acquired the ability to split water (H_2O) into hydrogen (H) and oxygen (O_2). This chemical reaction initiated the release of oxygen into the atmosphere. Owing to oxygen's toxicity, which was probably generated by free radicals, the increased levels of atmospheric oxygen led to the extinction of many anaerobic organisms.

This important atmospheric chemical event forced anaerobic organisms to acquire antioxidant systems to protect against damage produced by free radicals. Those that succeeded in developing protective antioxidant systems survived and ultimately evolved into multicellular organisms, including humans, who utilize oxygen for survival. Today, the amount of oxygen in dry air is about 21 percent; in water it is approximately 34 percent. We humans today have complex antioxidant systems that protect us from free radical damage. This antioxidant system, together with our immune system, protects us against toxic products of inflammation as well as from the release of glutamate. Glutamate is a neurotransmitter that kills neurons by excitotoxicity. Thus, it is detrimental to the brain.

Antioxidant systems in humans consist of two different components: antioxidant enzymes on the one hand, and dietary and endogenous antioxidant chemicals on the other. The first group includes

---

*However, an increase in short-term oxidative stress, such as seen during viral or bacterial infection, may be important in killing invading organisms, but it can also damage normal tissue.

glutathione peroxidase, catalase, and superoxide dismutase (SOD). The second group includes vitamin A, carotenoids, vitamin C, vitamin E, glutathione, alpha-lipoic acid, coenzyme Q10, L-carnitine, and polyphenolic compounds that are derived from plants, fruits, and vegetables. Antioxidant enzymes destroy free radicals by catalysis (the process of converting free radicals into nontoxic chemicals), whereas antioxidant chemicals destroy free radicals by scavenging them directly. Elevated levels of both components of the antioxidant system are essential for reducing oxidative stress optimally.

Free Radicals

Free radicals are atoms, molecules, or ions with unpaired electrons, which makes them highly reactive. Free radicals can damage deoxyribonucleic acid (DNA), ribonucleic acid (RNA), proteins, carbohydrates, and membranes. But these reactive oxygen species (ROS) also participate in cell-signaling systems that regulate growth, differentiation, and apoptosis of cells during the development and growth of humans.

The half-lives of free radicals vary from 10^{-9} seconds to days. This means that most are quickly destroyed after causing damage. For example, the half-life of hydroxyl free radicals is 10^{-9} seconds, superoxide anion's half-life is 10^{-5} seconds, and lipid peroxyl free radicals' half-life is 7 seconds. The half-life of nitric oxide is about one second, whereas the half-life of hydrogen peroxide is minutes. The half-life of semiquinone free radicals is days, and the half-lives of some organic free radicals are several days.

Free radicals can damage cells, but as mentioned above they also play an important role in the regulation of certain biochemical processes and the gene expressions necessary for our survival. Free radicals can be derived from oxygen as well as from nitrogen. In 1900 the first organic free radical, triphenylmethyl radical, was identified by Moses Gomberg of the University of Michigan. Free radicals are symbolized by a dot "•".

Types of Free Radicals

Several different types of free radicals derived from oxygen and nitrogen are generated in the body. The oxygen-derived free radicals include hydroxyl radical ($OH^•$), peroxyl radical ($ROO^•$), alkoxyl radical ($RO^•$), phenoxyl and semiquinone radicals ($ArO^•$, $HO-Ar-O^•$), and superoxide radical ($O^{•-}_2$). The nitrogen-derived free radicals include, NO, $^•ONOO^-$(peroxynitrite), and $^•NO_2$.

In addition to free radicals there are several oxidizing agents that are formed in the body. They include peroxynitrite, hydrogen peroxide, and lipid peroxide, all of which are very damaging to the cells.

Other radical species can also be formed by biological reactions in the body. For example, phenolic and other aromatic radical species can be formed during the metabolism of xenobiotic agents (agents that are foreign to the body). Furthermore, any antioxidant, when oxidized, can act as a free radical.

Sources of Free Radicals

The mechanism of free radical generation is very complex; therefore, it will be discussed in general terms here. Mitochondria are elongated membranous structures present in all cells in varying numbers; they use oxygen to produce energy. Most free radicals are produced in the mitochondria during energy generation, but some free radicals are also produced in the cytoplasm. During the process of generating energy, superoxide anions, hydroxyl radicals, and hydrogen peroxide are produced as by-products. It is estimated that approximately 2 percent of the oxygen consumed by the mitochondria remains partially unused. This unused oxygen leaks out of the mitochondria, thereby generating about 20 billion molecules of superoxide anions and hydrogen peroxide per cell per day.

During a bacterial or viral infection, phagocytic cells are activated. This activation generates high levels of nitric oxide, superoxide anions, and hydrogen peroxide within the infected cells in order that the infective agents are killed. An excessive production of free radicals by phagocytes can also damage normal cells and thereby can increase the risk that acute and/or chronic disease will develop.

It should also be noted that during the oxidative metabolism of fatty acids and other molecules in the body, free radicals are produced. Certain habits, such as the smoking of tobacco and the ingestion of some trace minerals such as free iron, copper, or manganese taken alone, can also increase the rate of production of free radicals in the body. Thus, the human body is exposed to different types and varying levels of free radicals on a daily basis.

The Formation of Free Radicals Derived from Oxygen and Nitrogen

The formative process of some reactive oxygen species (ROS: free radicals derived from oxygen) is described below.

When molecular oxygen (O_2) acquires an electron, the superoxide anion ($O_2{}^{\bullet-}$) is formed:

$$O_2 + e^- = O_2{}^{\bullet-}$$

Superoxide dismutase (SOD) and H^+ can react with $O_2{}^{\bullet-}$ to form hydrogen peroxide (H_2O_2):

$$2O_2{}^{\bullet-} + 2H^+ \text{ plus SOD} \rightarrow H_2O_2 + O_2$$
$$O_2{}^{\bullet-} + H^+ \rightarrow HO_2{}^{\bullet} \text{ (hydroperoxy radical)}$$
$$2HO_2{}^{\bullet} \rightarrow H_2O_2 + O_2$$

Ferric and ferrous forms of iron can react with superoxide anion and hydrogen peroxide to produce molecular oxygen (O_2) and hydroxyl radicals ($OH^{\bullet}$), respectively:

$$Fe^{3+} + O_2{}^{\bullet-} \rightarrow Fe^{2+} + O_2$$
$$Fe_2{}^+ + H_2O_2 \rightarrow Fe^{3+} + OH^{\bullet} + OH^- \text{ (Fenton reaction)}$$

Hydroxyl radicals can also be formed from superoxide anion by the Haber-Weiss reaction:

$$O_2^{\bullet-} + H_2O_2 \rightarrow O_2 + OH^- + OH^{\bullet}$$

Both the Fenton and Haber-Weiss reactions require a transition metal such as copper or iron. Among ROS, $OH^{\bullet}$ is the most damaging free radical and is very short-lived.

Hydroxyl radicals are very reactive with a variety of organic compounds, leading to the production of more radical compounds:

$$RH \text{ (organic compound)} + OH^{\bullet} \rightarrow R^{\bullet} \text{ (organic radical)} + H_2O$$
$$R^{\bullet} + O_2 \rightarrow RO_2^{\bullet} \text{ (peroxyl radical)}$$

For example, the DNA radical can be generated by reaction with a hydroxyl radical, and this can lead to a break in the DNA strand.

Catalase detoxifies hydrogen peroxide to form water and molecular oxygen:

$$H_2O_2 + \text{catalase} \rightarrow H_2O \text{ and } O_2$$

Reactive nitrogen species (RNS: free radicals derived from nitrogen) are represented by nitric oxide ($NO^{\bullet}$). NO is synthesized by the enzyme nitric oxide synthase from L-arginine. $NO^{\bullet}$ can combine with superoxide anion to form peroxynitrite, a powerful oxidant.

$$NO^{\bullet} + O_2^{\bullet-} \rightarrow ONOO^- \text{ (peroxynitrite)}$$

When protonated (likely at physiological pH), peroxynitrite spontaneously decomposes to reactive nitric dioxide and hydroxyl radicals:

$$ONOO^- + H^+ \rightarrow {}^{\bullet}NO_2 + OH^{\bullet}$$

Superoxide dismutase (SOD) can also enhance the peroxynitrite-mediated nitration of tyrosine residues on critical proteins, presumably via species similar to the nitronium cation (NO_2^+):

$$ONOO^- \text{ plus SOD} \rightarrow NO_2^+ \rightarrow \text{Nitration of tyrosine}$$

The Processes of Oxidation and Reduction

To fully comprehend the role of free radicals and antioxidants in the human body, it's important to grasp the relationship between the oxidation and reduction processes that are constantly taking place in the body.

Oxidation

Oxidation is a process wherein an atom or molecule gains oxygen or loses hydrogen or an electron. For example, carbon gains oxygen during oxidation and becomes carbon dioxide. Another example: A superoxide radical loses an electron during oxidation and becomes oxygen. Thus, an oxidizing agent is a molecule or atom that changes another chemical by adding oxygen to it or by removing an electron or hydrogen from it. Examples of oxidizing agents are free radicals, ozone, and ionizing radiation.

Reduction

Reduction is a process whereby an atom or molecule loses oxygen or gains hydrogen or an electron. For example, carbon dioxide loses oxygen and becomes carbon monoxide; carbon gains hydrogen and becomes methane; and oxygen gains an electron and becomes superoxide anion. Thus, a reducing agent is a molecule or atom that changes another chemical by removing oxygen from it or by adding an electron or hydrogen to it.

All antioxidants can be considered reducing agents. If there are more reduction processes taking place in the human body than oxidation processes, the body is apt to be maintained in a state of health. If, however, there are more oxidation processes than reduction processes transpiring, cellular injury, and eventually chronic neurodegenerative diseases such as Alzheimer's and Parkinson's, may develop.

Inflammation

Inflammation is a complex biological response initiated by the immune system, and as such it is one of the first responses of the immune system to infection. Inflammation in Latin is referred to as *inflammare,* or "setting on fire." When it occurs injured or infected cells release eicosanoids, cytokines, growth factors, and cytotoxic factors. These cytokines and other chemicals recruit immune cells to the site of infection so that the invading harmful organism can be eliminated and healing of the injured tissue can take place (Martin and Leibovich 2005). These recruited immune cells include white blood cells (leukocytes, macrophages, monocytes, lymphocytes, and plasma cells).

In the healing process injured tissue is replaced by a regeneration of native parenchymal cells (original cell type) or by the filling in of the injured site with fibroblastic tissue (scarring) or, most commonly, by a combination of both processes.

The primary features of inflammation at the affected site include redness and swelling. The site may also be warm to the touch and the afflicted individual may experience varying degrees of pain. These characteristics of inflammation were first recognized by Roman physician Cornelius Celsus (circa 30 BCE to 45 CE).

Types of Inflammation

Inflammation is divided into two categories: acute and chronic.

Acute inflammation occurs following cellular injury or infection by microorganisms. The period of acute inflammation is relatively short, typically lasting from a few minutes to a few days. The main features of acute inflammation are edema (an accumulation of exuded fluid and plasma in extracellular spaces) and the migration of leukocytes— primarily neutrophils—to the site of injury. Acute inflammation causes marked alterations in the blood vessels and invites inflammatory cells such as leukocytes to the site of injury. Subsequently, the leukocytes migrate to the site of injury by a process called chemotaxis. Leukocytes engulf pathogenic organisms by phagocytosis and kill them by generating bursts of reactive oxygen species and other toxic substances. Leukocytes can also engulf cellular debris and foreign antigens by a similar process and then degrade them with lysosomal proteolytic enzymes.

Leukocytes may also release excessive amounts of reactive oxygen species, pro-inflammatory cytokines, prostaglandins, adhesion molecules, and complement proteins, which can damage normal tissue.

An acute inflammatory reaction is tightly regulated and turned off soon after the injured sites are healed or the invading microbes removed. It is an absolutely essential process for removing both pathogens and cellular debris from the damaged site, thus allowing healing to occur. Acute inflammation, however, is effective only when the injurious stimuli or tissue damage is relatively mild. If the tissue damage is extensive or the levels of infective organisms are high, acute inflammatory reactions are not tuned off. Consequently the toxic products of these reactions can accelerate the rate of damage, which may result in organ failure and eventually even death.

Chronic inflammation occurs following persistent cellular injury or infection. The period of chronic inflammation is relatively lengthy and may last as long as the injury or infection exists. Persistent low-grade cellular injury, exposure to exogenous agents such as particulate silica, or infection can initiate chronic inflammation. Chronic inflammation is associated with most human neurodegenerative diseases such as Alzheimer's and Parkinson's, as well as mild traumatic brain injury (also called concussive injury) and post-traumatic stress disorders (PTSD).

In contrast to acute inflammation, which is characterized by vascular changes, edema, and primarily neutrophil infiltration, chronic inflammation is characterized by the presence of mononuclear cells. These mononuclear cells include macrophages, lymphocytes, and plasma cells. In the brain microglia cells, which represent inflammatory cells, become activated and migrate to the site of injury. During chronic inflammation the presence of angiogenesis and fibrosis can be observed at the site of injury.

Products of Inflammatory Reactions

As we know during inflammation several highly reactive agents are released. They may include cytokines, complement proteins, arachidonic acid (AA) metabolites, and endothelial/leukocyte adhesion molecules. They are briefly described below.

Cytokines are proteins released during both acute and chronic inflammation. They are produced by many cell types, primarily by activated lymphocytes and macrophages, but also by endothelium, epithelium, and connective tissue cells. In the brain cytokines are produced primarily by microglia cells, although some are produced by neurons. Pro-inflammatory cytokines include interleukin-6 (IL-6), IL-17, IL-18, IL-23, and tumor necrosis factor-alpha (TNF-alpha). These are all toxic to the cells. Anti-inflammatory cytokines also exist. They include IL-1, IL-4, IL-10, IL-11, and IL-13; they help in tissue repair at the site of injury.

If the tissue damage is severe, the pro-inflammatory cytokines may eclipse the repair function of the anti-inflammatory cytokines, thus participating in the progression of damage. Some pro-inflammatory cytokines such as IL-6 can also act as a neurotrophic factor. This means that it functions as a pro-inflammatory cytokine during the acute phase of injury and as a neurotrophic factor between the subacute and chronic phases of injury.

Cytokines are multifunctional, and individual cytokines may have both positive and negative regulatory actions. They also play an important role in modulating the functions of many other cell types. Cytokines mediate their action by binding to specific receptors on target cells. These receptors are regulated by exogenous and endogenous signals. Cytokines that regulate lymphocyte activation, growth, and differentiation include IL-2 and IL-4 (which favors growth), as well as IL-10 and transforming growth factor-beta (TGF-beta), which are negative regulators of immune responses. Cytokines involved with natural immunity include tumor necrosis factor-alpha (TNF-alpha), IL-1Beta, type I interferon (IFN-alpha and IFN-beta), and IL-6. Cytokines that activate inflammatory cells such as macrophages include IFN-gamma, TNF-alpha, TNF-beta, IL-5, IL-10, and IL-12. Cytokines that stimulate hematopoiesis (growth and differentiation of immature leukocytes) include IL-3, IL-7, c-kit ligand, granulocyte-macrophage colony-stimulating factor (GM-CSF), macrophage colony-stimulating factor (M-CSF), granulocyte CSF, and stem cell factor.

Chemokines are cytokines that stimulate leukocyte movement and direct them to the site of injury during inflammation. Many classical growth factors may also act as cytokines, and conversely, many cytokines exhibit activities of growth factors.

Complement Proteins: During inflammation twenty complement proteins, including their cleavage (degradation) products are released into the plasma. These proteins are the major humoral components of the innate immune response (Rus, Cudrici, and Niculescu 2005). When activated they can cause cell lysis (death) and exhibit proteolytic activity. They participate in both innate and adaptive immunity for protection against pathogenic organisms. Complement proteins are numbered C1 through C9, each of which has complex mechanisms of action on cells. Some of the complement proteins are also neurotoxic.

Arachidonic Acid (AA) Metabolites: Arachidonic acid is a 20-carbon fatty acid derived from dietary sources or formed from linoleic acid, which is an essential fatty acid. During inflammation AA metabolites (or eicosanoids) are released. These eicosanoids have diverse biological actions depending upon the cell type. The eicosanoids are synthesized by two major classes of enzymes: cyclooxygenase (COX) for the synthesis of prostaglandins and thromboxanes, and lipooxygenase for the synthesis of leukotrienes and lipoxins. There are two isoforms of cyclooxygenase: COX1 and COX2.

Endothelial/Leukocyte Adhesion Molecules: The immunoglobulin family molecules include two endothelial adhesion molecules: intracellular adhesion molecule-1 (ICAM-1) and vascular adhesion molecule-1 (VCAM-1). These adhesion molecules bind with leukocyte receptor integrins. They are induced by IL-1 and TNF-alpha. Both ICAM-1 and VCAM-1 are released during inflammatory reactions and have a diverse mechanism of action on cells.

CONCLUDING REMARKS

Approximately five million people in the United States suffer from the debilitating effects of Alzheimer's disease, which is the sixth leading cause of death in persons aged sixty-five and over. Over 500,000 senior citizens die from Alzheimer's and its complications every year. By 2050 the number of Americans over the age of sixty-five is estimated to be almost 89 million people. By this same year the anticipated cost to society of Alzheimer's is projected to be $1.2 trillion annually. At present it has no cure. All of these factors underscore the dire need to find treatment options that work in the prevention and enhanced management of this disease.

Research done to date indicates that increased oxidative stress and chronic inflammation in the body may be primary culprits responsible for the development of Alzheimer's disease. Increased oxidative stress is caused by the excessive production of free radicals derived from oxygen and nitrogen, which damages cells and tissues. Cell injury initiates an important biological event called inflammation, which is considered a protective response following infection with pathogenic organisms, exposure to antigens, and/or cellular damage. Inflammation is needed to kill invading pathogenic organisms and to remove cellular debris in order to facilitate the recovery process at the injured site.

The immune system is a highly complex, tightly regulated, biological response. Through the enactment of complex mechanisms, it plays an important defensive role against invading pathogenic organisms. Under certain conditions, however, the immune system can also produce toxic chemicals, which play an important role in the initiation and progression of chronic diseases, including neurodegenerative diseases such as Alzheimer's. Increased oxidative stress and chronic inflammation are associated with the initiation and progression of Alzheimer's. Therefore, attenuation of these two biological processes may reduce the risk of development and progression of this disease.

We will explore this supposition in the pages of this book. Now, though, let's have a look at the human brain, so we can better understand the anatomical configuration of this most complex organ of the human body and how the processes mentioned above may degrade its functions.

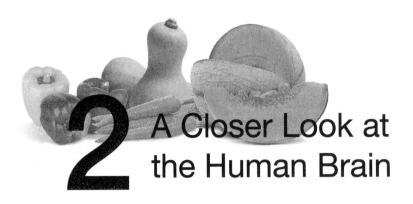

2 A Closer Look at the Human Brain

Despite extensive research by neuroanatomists, neurobiologists, neurochemists, and neurophysiologists, many aspects of the brain's structure and functioning remain tantalizingly unclear. The "Decade of the Brain," an initiative of the U.S. government in the 1990s under President George Bush, has increased our knowledge of brain functioning somewhat. Still, the work goes on to discover its myriad mysteries. Research endeavors include the study of animal and human neuronal and glial cell culture, the brain tissue of animals (primarily rodents and occasionally nonhuman primates), and human brains obtained at autopsy. Current research also includes noninvasive techniques such as electroencephalography (EEG), functional magnetic resonance imaging (fMRI), as well as invasive techniques such as obtaining fresh brain tissues from animals after euthanasia and human brain samples obtained at autopsy.

This chapter describes very briefly, and in simple terms, the structure and functions of the human brain that are relevant to chronic neurological diseases.

THE HUMAN BRAIN

Basic Facts

The average weight of the human adult brain is about three pounds (1.5 kg). In women the volume of the brain is approximately 1,130 cubic centimeters and in men it is about 1,260 cubic centimeters, although significant individual variations are found. The brain consists of three main regions: the forebrain, midbrain, and hindbrain. Brain regions are divided into the cerebrum, the cerebellum, the limbic system, and the brain stem.

The brain also contains four interconnected cavities that are filled with cerebrospinal fluid, as well as approximately 100 billion neurons. Neurons are a unique type of cell in that they can receive, synthesize, store, and transmit information from one neuron to another. Figure 2.1 presents a view of various structures of the human brain.

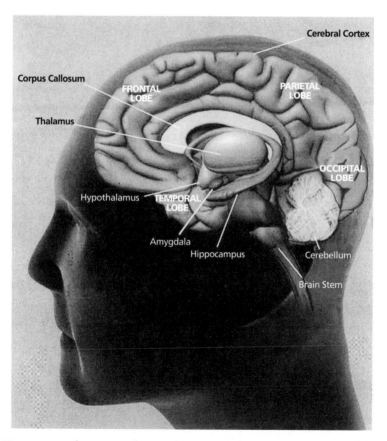

Figure 2.1. This image shows a horizontal slice of the head of an adult man, revealing the different structures of the human brain. Courtesy of the National Library of Medicine's Visible Human Project.

The Cerebrum and Its Function

The cerebrum or cortex is the largest part of the human brain, having a surface area of about 1.3 square feet (0.12 m2), folded in such a way so as to allow it to fit within the skull. This folding causes ridges of the cerebrum; these are called "gyri" collectively or "gyrus" in the singular. Crevices in the cortex are called "sulcus" or "sulci" (collectively). The cerebrum is divided into the right and left hemispheres, which are connected by a fibrous band of nerves called the corpus callosum. The corpus callosum is responsible for communication between the hemispheres. The right hemisphere controls the left side of the body and oversees temporal and spatial relationships, the analysis of nonverbal information, and the communication of emotion. The left hemisphere controls the right side of the body and produces and understands language.

The cortex of each hemisphere is divided into four lobes: the frontal lobe, the parietal lobe, the occipital lobe, and the temporal lobe. Certain functions of the lobes overlap with one another. The frontal lobe is responsible for cognition and memory, behavior, abstract thought processes, problem solving, analytic and critical reasoning, attention, creative thought, voluntary motor activity, language skills, emotional traits, intellect, reflection, judgment, physical reaction, inhibition, libido (the sexual urge), and initiative.

The parietal lobe oversees basic sensations such as touch, pain, pressure, temperature sensitivity, various joint movements, tactile sensations, spatial relationships and sensitivity to an exact point of tactile contact, as well as the ability to distinguish between two points of tactile stimulation, some language and reading functions, and some visual functions.

The occipital lobe is involved in interpreting visual impulses and reading.

The temporal lobe is involved with auditory (sound) sensations, speech, the sensation of smell, one's sense of identity, fear, music, some hearing, some vision pathways, and some emotions and memories.

Nerve cells form the gray surface of the cerebrum, which is a little thicker than the nerve fibers that carry signals between nerve cells and other parts of the body.

The Cerebellum

The cerebellum is much smaller than the cerebrum, but like the cerebrum, it has a highly folded surface. This portion of the brain is associated with the coordination of movement; posture and balance; and cardiac, respiratory, and vasomotor functions.

The Limbic System

The limbic system includes the thalamus, hypothalamus, amygdala, and hippocampus. It is responsible for processing emotion and storing and retrieving memory.

The Thalamus

The thalamus is a large, paired, egg-shaped structure containing clusters of nuclei (gray matter); it is responsible for sensory and motor functions. Sensory information enters the thalamus, which relays the information to the overlying cerebral cortex.

The Hypothalamus

The hypothalamus is located ventral to the thalamus and is responsible for regulating emotion, thirst, hunger, circadian rhythms, the autonomic nervous system, and the pituitary gland.

The Amygdala

The amygdala is located in the temporal lobe just beneath the surface of the hippocampus and is associated with memory, emotion, and fear.

The Hippocampus

The hippocampus is that portion of the cerebral hemisphere in the basal medial part of the temporal lobe. It is responsible for learning and memory. It is also responsible for converting short-term memory to more permanent memory and for recalling spatial relationships.

The Brain Stem

The brain stem is located underneath the limbic system. It's responsible for regulating breathing, heartbeat, and blood pressure. The main constituents of the brain stem are the midbrain, pons, medulla, and the pyramidal and extrapyramidal systems.

The Midbrain

The midbrain, also called the mesencephalon, is located between the forebrain and the hindbrain (pons and medulla), and includes the tectum and the tegmentum. The midbrain participates in regulating motor functions, eye movements, pupil dilation, and hearing. The midbrain also contains the crus cerebri, which is made up of nerve fibers. These nerve fibers connect the cerebral hemispheres to the cerebellum and substantia nigra. The substantia nigra neurons are pigmented and consist of two parts, the pars reticulate and the pars compacta. Nerve cells of the pars compacta contain dark pigments (melanin granules). These neurons synthesize dopamine and project to either the caudate nucleus or the putamen. Both the caudate nucleus and the putamen are part of the basal ganglia, which regulate movement and coordination. The striatum part of the brain consists of the globus pallidus, the substantia nigra, and the basal ganglia.

The Pons

The pons (metencephalon) is located below the posterior portion of the cerebrum and above the medulla oblongata. It regulates arousal and sleep and participates in controlling autonomic functions. It also relays sensory information between the cerebrum and the cerebellum.

The Medulla (Medulla Oblongata)

The medulla, also called the myelencephalon, is the lower portion of the brain stem and is located anterior to the cerebellum. It regulates autonomic functions and relays nerve signals between the brain and the spinal cord.

The Pyramidal and Extrapyramidal Systems

Both the pyramidal and the extrapyramidal systems represent part of the motor pathways within the brain stem. Neurons of the pyramidal system have no synapses, whereas neurons of the extrapyramidal system have synapses. Nerve fibers of the pyramidal system originate in the cerebral cortex and continue on to the thalamus and medulla oblongata. The pyramidal system regulates fine movements such as control of the jaws, lips, and aspects of the face, conscious thoughts, and movements of the hands and fingers.

The major parts of the extrapyramidal system include the red nucleus, the caudate nucleus, the putamen, the substantia nigra, the globus pallidus, and the subthalamic nuclei. The extrapyramidal system dampens erratic motions, maintains muscle tone, and allows for overall functional stability.

Other Components of the Brain

Basal Ganglia

The basal ganglia is located deep in the cerebral hemisphere. It consists of the caudate nucleus, the putamen, the globus pallidus, the substantia nigra, and the subthalamic nucleus. It regulates posture and emotion, such as happiness, through dopamine. It also regulates movements and their intensity.

Neurons

Neurons (nerve cells) in the brain are highly complex, specialized cells that receive information, process it, and then send it in the form of electrical impulses through synapses to other neurons. (Synapses connect a neuron to other neurons.) A diagrammatic representation of a neuron is provided in figure 2.2. The estimation of the number of neurons in the brain varies from study to study, with one study estimating that the human brain contains about 100 billion neurons and about 100 trillion synapses (Williams and Herrup 1988). Approximately 3 to 5 percent of neurons are lost from the brain every decade after the age of thirty-five. Therefore, it's possible that older individuals may have fewer neurons than the aforementioned estimated 100 billion neurons.

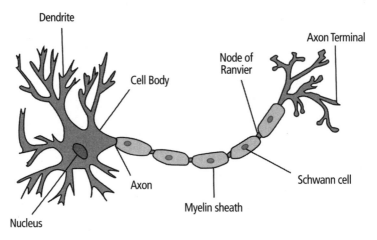

Figure 2.2. A typical neuron

A neuron consists of the cell body, (also called soma), dendrites, and an axon. The cell body contains a nucleus, mitochondria, Golgi bodies, and lysosomes, as well as smooth and rough endoplasmic reticulum. Dendrites are filamentous structures that extend away from the cell body. They branch into several processes that become thinner the further they extend. An axon is also a filamentous structure that extends itself from the cell body at a swelling called the axon hillock, which branches away from the soma. As it extends further it undergoes further branching at the axonal terminal. These branches, through synapses, can communicate with more than one neuron at a time.

The soma can have numerous dendrites, but only one axon. The axons of presynaptic neurons contain mitochondria and microtubules. The microtubules help to transport neurotransmitters from the cytoplasm to the tip of the axon where they're stored in very small vesicles.

Incoming synaptic signals from other neurons are received by the dendrites; the outgoing signals are sent through the axons.

Presynaptic neurons are those that transmit signals to different neurons through the axon and its synapses. The neurons that receive these signals are called postsynaptic neurons. Axon terminals contain neurotransmitters that are released at the postsynaptic neurons.

There are three major specialized neurons: sensory neurons, motor neurons, and interneurons. Sensory neurons respond to touch, sound, light, and many other stimuli. They affect the cells of sensory organs and then send signals to the brain and the spinal cord. Motor neurons receive signals from the brain and the spinal cord, cause muscle contractions, and affect glands. Interneurons connect neurons to other neurons within the same regions of the brain.

Other neurons include cholinergic neurons, dopaminergic neurons, glutamatergic neurons, GABAergic neurons, and serotonergic neurons. They are described below.

Cholinergic neurons: Cholinergic neurons are primarily located in the basal forebrain, striatum, and cerebral cortex. Each neuron contains an enzyme choline acetyltransferase, which makes the neurotransmitter acetylcholine from choline. Acetylcholine is degraded by another enzyme called acetylcholinesterase. Acetylcholine is stored in small vesicles in the nerve endings. An elevation of extracellular calcium causes the release of acetylcholine from the vesicles. The action of this neurotransmitter is mediated through nicotinic receptors and muscarinic receptors. Cholinergic neurons are the primary source of acetylcholine for the cerebral cortex; acetylcholine regulates memory and learning ability. A loss of cholinergic neurons is associated with some neurodegenerative diseases, including dementia with or without Alzheimer's disease.

Dopaminergic neurons: Dopamine belongs to the group of catecholamines. It is degraded by the enzyme catechol-O-methyltransferase

(COMT). Neurons that produce dopamine (dopaminergic neurons) are also referred to as dopamine (DA) neurons. Dopaminergic neurons make a neurotransmitter dopamine (3,4-dihydrxyphenethylamine) from L-DOPA (L-3,4-dihydroxyphenylalanine) with the help of the enzyme DOPA decarboxylase. L-dopa is made from the amino acid tyrosine by the enzyme tyrosine hydroxylase. Dopamine neurons are primarily located in the substantia nigra pars compacta, a part of the basal ganglia present in the midbrain. This area of the brain also contains melanin granules and a high level of iron (Chinta and Andersen 2005). The presence of melanin granules and iron exposes dopamine neurons to increased levels of free radicals.

The ventral tegmental area of the midbrain also contains dopamine neurons, which send their projections to the striatum, globus pallidus, and subthalamic nucleus. Although the number of dopamine neurons is relatively less, they regulate several functions, including voluntary movement, mood reward addiction, stress, motivation, arousal, and sexual gratification. The action of dopamine is mediated via dopamine receptors D1-5. Dopamine is converted to norepinephrine by the enzyme dopamine B-carboxylase and norepinephrine is converted to epinephrine by the enzyme phenylethanolamine-N-methyltransferase. Catecholamines (dopamine, norepinephrine, and epinephrine) are degraded by the enzyme COMT and/or monoamine oxidase. A loss of dopamine neurons is associated with Parkinson's disease.

Glutamatergic neurons: Neurons producing glutamate are called glutamatergic neurons. Glutamate is considered one of the most important neurotransmitters for proper brain functioning. As mentioned earlier it is considered excitatory because it causes hyperactivity and kills neurons by excitotoxicity. Excitotoxicity refers to the ability of glutamate to kill neurons by producing prolonged excitatory synaptic transmission. Glutamate mediates its actions through its receptors N-methyl-D-aspartate (NMDA), a-amino-3-hydroxy-5-methyl-4-isoxazolepropionic acid (AMPA), kianate, and G-protein coupled glutamate receptors (mGLuR1).

Glutamate is a nonessential amino acid that does not cross the blood-brain barrier. It is made in the neurons from glutamine that is present in the synaptic terminal. Glutamine is released from glial cells and accumulates in the presynaptic terminal where it is converted to glutamate by the mitochondrial enzyme glutaminase. Glutamate is stored in very small vesicles and is released from these vesicles by the glutamate transporters present in glial cells and presynaptic terminals. Glutamate is converted back to glutamine by the enzyme glutamine synthetase, which is present in glial cells. Glutamine is then transported from the glial cells to presynaptic nerve terminals.

More than half of the brain synapses release glutamate. Following brain injury, glutamate is released and accumulates in the extracellular space of the brain. This is responsible for the neurodegeneration that is commonly found in some neurodegenerative diseases. An increase in the extracellular levels of glutamate in the brain is associated with some neurological diseases, such as traumatic brain injury, post-traumatic stress disorder (PTSD), and Huntington's disease.

GABAergic neurons: Neurons producing gamma-aminobutyric acid (GABA) are called GABAergic neurons. As opposed to the excitatory function of glutamate, GABA exhibits inhibitory transmission and thereby balances the effect of glutamate on the neurons. It's been estimated that about 25 percent of neurons in the cortex use GABA (Tamminga et al. 2004). Like glutamate, GABA does not cross the blood-brain barrier. It is made in the neuron from glutamate by the enzyme L-glutamic acid decarboxylase and converted back to glutamate by a metabolic process called GABA shunt. The first step in the GABA shunt is to convert α-ketoglutarate into L-glutamic acid by the enzyme GABA α-oxoglutarate transaminase. Glutamic acid decarboxylase (GAD) converts glutamic acid into GABA.

Like glutamate, GABA is a nonessential amino acid. It mediates its action through GABA receptors (GABAa and GABAb). GABAa receptors regulate rapid mood changes as well as fear and anxiety.

These receptors are the target for sedative drugs such as alcohol, benzodiazepines, and barbiturates. GABAb receptors regulate memory and depressed moods and pain. Stimulation of this receptor can reduce the release of dopamine that would inhibit the reward response induced by external agents such recreational drugs.

Purkinje neurons are the largest neurons, and they belong to the class of GABA neurons that are located in the cortex of the cerebellum. They can have over 1,000 dendritic branches. One Purkinje neuron can make connections with several neurons. These neurons possess a bidirectional signaling axis, which produces inhibitory as well as excitatory interneurons that play an important role in motor learning and general learning ability (Fleming et al. 2013).

Serotonergic neurons: Neurons producing serotonin (5HT-2) are called serotonergic neurons. Serotonergic neurons are located in the raphe nuclei of the midbrain, pons, and medulla; they also accumulate in the synaptic clefts. The levels of serotonin in the synaptic cleft depend on the synthesis as well as the reuptake of serotonin. Serotonin neurons send projections to the cortex and basal ganglia.

Serotonin (5-hydroxytryptamine) is made from the amino acid tryptophan by the enzymes tryptophan hydroxylase and tryptophan decarboxylase. Serotonin does not cross the blood-brain barrier; however, L-tryptophan and its metabolite 5-hydroxytryptophan can enter the blood-brain barrier and increase the brain's level of serotonin. Serotonin mediates its action through serotonin receptors (5HT-1 and 5HT-2). It regulates mood, appetite, sleep, and, to some extent, memory and learning ability.

Glial Cells

Glial cells are totally different from nerve cells. Characterized by the presence of glial fibrillary acidic protein (GFAP), which is specific to them, they're considered supporting cells for the development, survival, and synaptic functions of neurons. They also help in the repair processes after an injury to the brain. Like neurons, they don't divide in the adult brain, but unlike neurons, they rapidly divide in response to brain injury. They do not have axons or elaborate neurites. The number of glial cells in the brain is much higher than the number of nerve cells. Indeed, the glial cells' main role is to support the nerve cells and to ensure their proper functioning. (The term "glial" is derived from the Greek word for "glue.") There are three types of glial cells in mature human brains: astrocytes, oligodendrocytes, and microglia cells.

Astrocytes: Astrocytes have small cytoplasmic processes that give an appearance of stars. They remove excess neurotransmitters released from nerve terminals and thereby regulate synaptic transmission. These cells also help to maintain concentrations of calcium and potassium in the brain.

Oligodendrocytes: Oligodendrocytes produce myelin, which wraps around the axons of neurons. The myelin sheath of oligodendrocytes forms electrical insulation around the nerve fibers and thereby facilitates rapid transmission of electrical signals in the brain.

Microglia: Microglia cells are smaller in size and are considered immune cells of the brain. In response to cellular injury the microglia migrate to the site of injury to help in the healing processes. These cells also produce pro-inflammatory cytokines that can damage neurons if the injury persists.

Growth Factors

Brains produce growth factors, which include nerve growth factor (NGF), brain-derived neurotrophic factor (BDNF), and glial cell-derived neurotrophic factor (GDNF). These growth factors are important in the development, survival, and regeneration of neurons following an injury. Both astrocytes and embryonic neurons from the mouse brain produce nerve growth factor in culture. The levels of nerve growth factor were higher in the growth phase than in the nongrowth phase. Unlike astrocytes, embryonic neurons continue to produce nerve growth factor during the nongrowth phase (Houlgatte et al. 1989). It has been demonstrated that the presence of both glial cell-derived neurotrophic factor and brain-derived neurotrophic factor is required for the survival of certain neurons, including dopamine neurons (Erickson, Brosenitsch, and Katz 2001). Brain-derived neurotrophic factors act via their respective receptors.

Decreased levels of brain-derived neurotrophic factor are associated with Alzheimer's disease. It has been demonstrated that acute aerobic exercise increased plasma levels of brain-derived neurotrophic factor in patients with Alzheimer's disease as well as in healthy individuals (Coelho et al. 2014).

In a clinical study of ninety-one teenagers, it was demonstrated that serum levels of brain-derived neurotrophic factor increased after exercise and improved cognitive function (Lee et al. 2014).

The level of basic fibroblastic growth factor (bFGF) increases in glioma cells. It has been demonstrated that insertion of basic fibroblastic growth factor into astrocytes causes a migration and proliferation of cells without tumor formation (Holland and Varmus 1998). This observation suggests that increased levels of basic fibroblastic growth factor are not related to cancer formation in glial cells. An elevation of basic fibroblastic growth factor may be a signal for the astrocytes to divide.

Neurotransmitters

Neurotransmitters are chemicals produced in the neurons and are located primarily at the synapses. They carry signals from one neuron to another; these signals may be inhibitory or excitatory. Neurotransmitters are released in response to a specific stimulus; all have different functions. Electric charges from the cytoplasm of the neurons release neurotransmitters and send them across the synapse. They travel through the gap junction to bind with the receptors specific to a particular neurotransmitter located on the surface of postsynaptic neurons.

Synapses

A synapse is the junction between two neurons (presynaptic neurons and postsynaptic neurons). The gap between two neurons is about 0.02 microns.

Processes of the Brain

Conduction of Signals

In order to communicate neurons send electrical signals (action potential) to other neurons through the axons. This process of sending electrical signals is called conduction. An electrical signal is formed when ions, which are electrically charged particles, move across the neuronal membrane. The movement of ions takes place through ion channels that can open or close in the presence of neurotransmitters. The neuronal membrane is normally at rest (in a polarized state). The influx and outflux of ions through ion channels during neurotransmission depolarizes the target neuron. When this depolarization reaches a point of no return (threshold), a large electrical signal is generated. This electrical signal propagates along the axon until it reaches the axon terminal where the conduction of the electrical signal ends. The neuron then sends its output to other neurons.

Synaptic Transmission (Neurotransmission)

Synaptic transmission between neurons occurs by the movement of an electric or chemical signal across a synapse. At the electrical synapse the electrical signals are considered output, whereas at the chemical synapse neurotransmitters are considered output. At the electrical synapses two neurons are physically connected to each other through the gap junction that we mentioned earlier. The gap junction allows changes in the electrical signal of one neuron to affect the other. Chemical synaptic neurotransmission occurs at the chemical synapse. In this type of transmission the presynaptic neurons and the postsynaptic neurons are separated by the synaptic cleft. The synaptic cleft allows signals coming from one neuron to pass to another neuron.

CONCLUDING REMARKS

The human brain is the body's most complex organ about which much is still unknown. It's composed of approximately 100 billion neurons and 100 trillion synapses that extend over three areas: the forebrain, midbrain, and hindbrain. Parts of the brain include the cerebrum, the cerebellum, the limbic system, and the brain stem. Four cavities filled with cerebrospinal fluid are also part of the brain.

Brain cells include the neurons mentioned above, as well as glial cells. Neurons, both presynaptic and postsynaptic, hold and transmit information via the synapses in a process known as conduction. There are many different types of brain neurons; each type has a different function. Chemicals that transport signals from neuron to neuron, called neurotransmitters, are also part of the picture. Glial cells support the neurons and help to heal the brain in the case of brain injury. Substances called "growth factors" are produced by the brain and help neurons to recover following brain injury.

Now that we understand a little bit more about how the brain actually works, let's look at how oxidative stress and inflammation may impact upon it in the development and progression of Alzheimer's disease.

3 Oxidative Stress and Inflammation and Related Alzheimer's Studies

In this book I propose a unified hypothesis that increased oxidative stress and chronic inflammation are primarily responsible for the initiation and progression of Alzheimer's disease. In this chapter I will expand upon this hypothesis and then examine the results of studies done that pertain to this issue. It's not just oxidative stress and inflammation that play a role in Alzheimer's disease, however. There are risk factors, both internally generated and external, which may be involved as well. Let's examine some of them here, before moving on to a closer examination of oxidative stress and inflammation.

FACTORS THAT IMPACT ON THE DEVELOPMENT OF ALZHEIMER'S DISEASE

There are many agents that can increase the risk of developing Alzheimer's disease, and there are some factors that may decrease the risk. Factors that can increase the risk include external factors (environment-, diet- and lifestyle-related) as well as the internal factors of increased oxidative stress, mitochondrial dysfunction, chronic inflammation, and increased levels of beta-amyloids (Aß1-42 peptides generated from APP), increased cholesterol levels, and proteasome inhibition. In addition, mutations in APP, presenilin-1, and presenilin-2 genes increase the risk of familial Alzheimer's disease.

Factors that may decrease the risk include exercise and vitamins. Let's look at them next.

External Agents That May Decrease the Risk of Developing Alzheimer's

Exercise

The injection of beta-amyloids directly into the brain caused cognitive dysfunction (memory loss), increased oxidative stress, and inflammation in male Swiss albino mice. However, exercise prevented memory loss, oxidative stress, and inflammation in these mice (Souza et al. 2013). The relevance of these observations in humans is not known.

Vitamins

It has been reported that a high dietary intake of vitamin C and vitamin E may reduce the risk of Alzheimer's, and among current cigarette smokers the intake of beta-carotene and flavonoids may also decrease the risk of Alzheimer's (Engelhart et al. 2002).

External Agents That May Increase the Risk of Developing Alzheimer's

Studies on the impacts of environmental-, dietary-, and lifestyle-related factors on the risk of developing Alzheimer's are important in identifying agents that may prevent it. Several such agents have been identified by survey-types of studies (epidemiologic studies) in humans. They include the following:

Environmental Factors

Exposure to aluminum: A high consumption of aluminum from drinking water may increase the risk of developing dementia (Rondeau et al. 2009).

Exposure to electromagnetic fields: The growing use of electromagnetic field (EMF) technology has raised concerns about its potentially adverse, long-term health effects. This includes concerns about electromagnetic pulse (EMP), which is one type of widely used EMF technology. Exposure to electromagnetic fields may produce beneficial or harmful effects as regards memory loss, depending on the strength of the electromagnetic field. This has been demonstrated in experimental models of study, an example of which is presented here.

An electromagnetic pulse (EMP) is a burst of electromagnetic energy. The exposure of healthy male rats to 100, 1,000, and 10,000 pulses of EMP induced memory loss, which was correlated with increased beta-amyloid production. This exposure was also associated with increases in beta-amyloid oligomer (binding of less than four units of beta-amyloids), amyloid precursor protein (APP), and decreased antioxidant enzyme superoxide dismutase (SOD) activity, as well as decreased glutathione levels in the nerve cells (Jiang et al. 2013).

Exposure of male mice to 200 pulses of EMP increased lipid peroxidation but reduced the activities of the antioxidant enzymes SOD, glutathione peroxidase, and catalase, as well as the levels of glutathione. It was also found that exposure to EMP decreased the learning ability of mice (Chen et al. 2011).

These results suggest that EMP at lower EMF field strengths induces memory loss and learning disability by increasing oxidative stress. In contrast to the effects of EMP at lower EMF field strengths in normal mice, in Alzheimer's transgenic (Tg) old mice, long-term exposure to high-strength EMF (918 MHz) improved memory function and reduced beta-amyloid-induced damage to nerve cells in the brain (Arendash et al. 2012).

Exposure to chronic noise: Exposure of rats to chronic noise may induce biochemical changes in the brain such as are found in Alzheimer's disease. For example, exposure to chronic noise increased the levels of hyperphosphorylated tau protein (P-tau) and neurofibrillary tangles in the brain of male Wistar rats (Cui et al. 2012).

Dietary Factors

Vitamin D deficiency: Vitamin D deficiency appears to be associated with both Alzheimer's disease and Parkinson's disease (Evatt et al. 2008).

It has been demonstrated that a high-fat/high-cholesterol diet induced a loss of working memory and caused inflammation and increased production of beta-amyloids in mice (Thirumangalakudi et al. 2008).

Following a high-fat/high-colesterol diet also enhanced the levels of hyperphosphorylated tau protein (P-tau) and reduced the levels of postsynaptic protein, which reduces the survival and function of the synapses (Bhat and Thirumangalakudi 2013).

Lifestyle-related Factors

Cigarette smoking: Cigarette smoking is considered a risk factor for developing Alzheimer's disease. A study showed that exposure to cigarette smoke increased the levels of oxidative stress in the hippocampus region of rats compared to those not exposed to cigarette smoke (Ho et al. 2012).

Exposure to smoke also reduced the normal functioning of the synapses. In addition, exposure to cigarette smoke decreased the levels of acetylated-tubulin and increased the levels of phosphorylated tau protein in the hippocampus region of the brain. It also increased the rate of production and the accumulation of beta-amyloids in the neurons. Exposure to cigarette smoke increased markers of oxidative stress and proinflammatory cytokines in the brain of Lewis rats compared to control animals that were not exposed to cigarette smoke (Khanna et al. 2013).

The relevance of observations made on external agents that increase or decrease the risk of developing Alzheimer's in humans is not known.

Nevertheless, minimizing one's exposure to agents that increase the risk of Alzheimer's disease and adopting those agents and practices that reduce the risk of it could be useful in reducing its incidence.

Internal Factors That May Increase the Risk of Developing Alzheimer's Disease

The major internal factors that increase the risk of developing Alzheimer's and enhance its progression include increased oxidative stress, mitochondrial dysfunction, chronic inflammation, increased production of beta-amyloids (Aß1-42 peptides) from amyloid precursor protein (APP), and increased levels of cholesterol, proteasome inhibition, and mutations in APP, presenilin-1 and presenilin-2 genes. Among these internal risk factors, increased oxidative stress appears to be one of the earliest biochemical defects initiating damage to the nerve cells in the brain of Alzheimer's patients (Prasad and Bondy 2014).

The other risk factors—mitochondrial dysfunction, chronic inflammation, increased production of beta-amyloids, increased levels of cholesterol, and proteasome inhibition—occur subsequent to increased oxidative stress. The cumulative impact of these factors increases the underlying oxidative stress and, together with other biochemical and genetic risk factors, contributes to the development and progression of Alzheimer's disease. These internal risk factors provide useful targets to be utilized in the development of a rational strategy for the prevention and improved management of this disease.

In terms of the biochemical and genetic factors (referenced above) that play an important role in the development and progression of Alzheimer's disease, please see the review that pertains to this, which I am a co-author of (Prasad, Cole, and Prasad 2002).

Impact of Free Radicals on the Brain

Although we discussed free radicals in the previous chapter, we will expand on that discussion here. Let's take a closer look at them, specifically in regard to how they contribute to oxidative stress in the brain.

The human brain represents only 5 percent of body weight, but it utilizes about 25 percent of the respired oxygen we breathe. Free radicals are generated by mitochondria in the brain during the processing of oxygen to water, during infection, and during normal oxidative metabolism (biological processes requiring oxygen for degradation of certain compounds or for their conversion to active compounds). The use of oxygen by the mitochondria is essential in producing energy, and generally mitochondria are the major source of free radicals. (However, some free radicals are produced outside the mitochondria in the cytoplasm.) Mitrochondria that have been damaged by free radicals produce more free radicals.

During normal aerobic exercises the mitochondria of one rat nerve cell will process about 10^{12} (one trillion) oxygen molecules and reduce them to water. During this process free radicals such as superoxide anion ($O_2^{-\bullet}$), hydrogen peroxide (H_2O_2), and hydroxyl ($OH^\bullet$) are formed. As mentioned previously, during bacterial or viral infection, phagocytic cells of the immune system generate high levels of nitric oxide (NO), $O_2^{-\bullet}$, and H_2O_2 in order to kill infective agents; however, these free radicals can also damage normal cells (Ames et al. 1973). During the degradation of fatty acids and other molecules by peroxisomes, H_2O_2 is produced as a by-product. During the oxidative metabolism of ingested toxins, free radicals are also generated.

Some brain enzymes such as monoamine oxidase (MAO), tyrosine hydroxylase, and L-amino acid oxidase produce H_2O_2 as a normal by-product of their activity (Coyle and Puttfarcken 1993). Furthermore, auto-oxidation of ascorbate and catecholamines (neurotransmitters) generates free radicals and H_2O_2 in the brain (Graham 1978).

Oxidative stress can also be generated by calcium-mediated activation of the glutamate receptor N-methyl-D-aspartate (NMDA) (Chan and Fishman 1980).

Another free radical, nitric oxide (NO), is formed by the enzyme nitric oxide synthase stimulated by calcium. Nitric oxide can react with superoxide anion $O_2^{-\bullet}$ to form peroxynitrite, which then can form $OH^\bullet$, the highly reactive hydroxyl free radical. Stimulation of the NMDA receptor elevated the levels of free radicals ($O_2^{-\bullet}$ and $OH^{\bullet}$) (Lafon-Cazal et al. 1993). Some enzymes, such as xanthine oxidase and flavoprotein oxidase (e.g., aldehyde oxidase), also form superoxide anions during metabolism of their respective substrates. Oxidation of hydroquinone and thiols and synthesis of uric acid from purines form superoxide anions. These free radicals are produced outside the mitochondria.

Certain external agents can increase oxidative stress in the body. For example, cigarette smoking increases the level of nitric oxide (NO) (Kiyosawa et al. 1990; Reznick et al. 1992) and depletes antioxidant levels (Schectman, Byrd, and Hoffmann 1991; Duthie, Arthur, and James 1991).

Free iron and copper can increase the levels of free radicals (Winterbourn 1995), and plant-derived antioxidants such as phenolic compounds (chlorogenic and caffeic acid) can be oxidized to form free radicals (Ames, Profet, and Gold 1990). These studies suggest that the brain generates high levels of free radicals every day. In addition to high levels of free radical production, the brain is the organ of the body that has the highest levels of unsaturated fatty acids; these are easily damaged by free radicals. Paradoxically, the brain is least prepared to handle this excessive load (of free radicals), because it has low levels of both antioxidant enzymes and dietary and endogenous antioxidants. These inherent biological features make the brain very vulnerable to damage produced by free radicals.

Despite this, the clinical symptoms of Alzheimer's disease may appear in some individuals only after the age of sixty-five when the large number of neurons responsible for storing and recalling memory is lost. This later onset is due to the fact that neurons exhibit a high degree of plasticity (the capacity to perform normal function with fewer nerve cells). The ability of surviving neurons to compensate function for the lost neurons may have developed in response to the increased oxidative environment of the brain, which causes a gradual loss of neurons.

As discussed earlier but bears repeating here, the types of

oxygen-derived free radicals include superoxide anion ($O_2^{-\bullet}$), and hydroxyl radical ($OH^\bullet$), hydroperoxy radical ($HO_2^\bullet$), organic radical ($R^\bullet$), peroxy radical ($RO_2^\bullet$), and H_2O_2.

Reactive nitrogen species (RNS) are represented by nitric oxide ($NO^\bullet$). NO is synthesized by the enzyme nitric oxide synthase from L-arginine, and in the brain it acts both as a neurotransmitter and, in excessive amounts, as a neurotoxin. $NO^\bullet$ can combine with superoxide anion to form peroxynitrite, a powerful oxidant. Reactive nitric oxide ($^\bullet NO_2$) is also formed.

These data reveal that several different types of radicals are constantly formed in the brain. Their levels can be increased by an enhanced turnover of catecholamines, increased levels of free iron, impaired mitochondrial functions, as well as decreased glutathione levels.

Antioxidant enzymes, which protect nerve cells against the damaging effects of these free radicals, include catalase, superoxide dismutase (SOD), and glutathione peroxidase. Correspondingly, decreased levels of catalase, glutathione peroxidase, or SOD can increase the amount of free radicals present in the brain. Consumption of a diet low in antioxidants may also increase these free radical levels. Thus, maintaining a healthy balance of antioxidants in the body is essential for proper brain functioning.

STUDIES DONE

Extensive studies on animal models of Alzheimer's disease and cell-culture model of Alzheimer's further indicate that increased oxidative stress may be one of the earliest defects that initiate damage to the nerve cells in the brain of Alzheimer's patients. Because of the increased production of free radicals and reduced levels of antioxidants, the brain is particularly sensitive to free radical damage. The diagram in the box below is a representation of the various pathways of increased oxidative stress in the brains of patients with Alzheimer's disease, which causes the death of the nerve cells therein.

Pathways of Oxidative Stress in Causing Neuronal Death in Alzheimer's Patients

Increased oxidative stress→→beta-secretase elevation→→ gamma-secretase elevation→→APP cleavage→→beta-amyloid elevation→→aggregation of beta-amyloids by copper and zinc→→produce free radicals→→death of nerve cells

Increased oxidative stress→→mitochondrial dysfunction→→ Reduced production of energy→→increased production of free radicals→→death of nerve cells

Increased oxidative stress→→activation of microglia cells→→production of pro-inflammatory cytokines and free radicals→→death of nerve cells

Increased oxidative stress→→inhibited proteasome activity→→ accumulation of misfolded proteins (hyperphosphorylated tau and APOE)→→participation in the formation of NFT→→ death of nerve cells

Increased oxidative stress→→tau hyperphosphorylation→→ formation of oligomer of phosphorylated tau→→ disruption of synaptic function→→loss of synapses→→ death of nerve cells

Mutation in APP, PS-1, and PS-2 genes*→→increased production of beta-amyloids→→increased production of free radicals→→ death of nerve cells

---

*"PS-1" is presenilin-1, and "PS-2" is presenilin-2.

Animal Studies

Sufficient energy is needed for the synapses of the nerve cells to survive and function properly. In a person with Alzheimer's disease, reduced energy due to defects in mitochondrial function may account for the loss of the proper functioning of these synapses. Using a transgenic mouse model of Alzheimer's (APP23 mice), it was demonstrated that reduced energy production and increased protein oxidation occur in the cortex of mice that were asymptomatic for Alzheimer's disease. This suggests that increased oxidative stress occurs prior to the development of other biochemical and genetic defects that contribute to the formation of increased levels of beta-amyloids, senile plaques, and neurofibrillary tangles (Hartl et al. 2012).

Using an imaging technique on the brain of transgenic mice in the Alzheimer's model, it was shown that increased oxidative stress preceded the activation of the enzyme caspase, which led to the death of nerve cells within twenty-four hours (Xie et al. 2013).

Transgenic A mice (tau 3xTg) exhibited memory loss and fear. Pretreatment of these animals with a SOD/catalase mimetic (producing the same effect as SOD or catalase), EUK-207, prevented memory loss and fear. It also reduced the levels of beta-amyloids, tau, and hyperphosphorylated tau proteins, oxidized nucleic acid, and lipid peroxidation in the amygdala and hippocampus regions of the brain (Clausen et al. 2012).

These results suggest that increased oxidative stress occurs prior to other biochemical defects in the initiation of damage to the nerve cells. This is further supported by the fact that pretreatment of transgenic Alzheimer's mice with an antioxidant prevented damages associated with the degeneration of nerve cells and improved the symptoms of the disease.

Cell-Culture Studies

Using primary neuron cultures from normal, newborn mice and transgenic mice expressing mutated APP and mutated presenilin-1, it was demonstrated that markers of oxidative stress, such as oxidized protein, 4-hydroxynonenal (4-HNE), and 3-nitrotyrosine (3-NT) were elevated and mitochondrial functions were impaired in these nerve cells compared to those nerve cells obtained from normal mice (Sompol et al.

2008). This study suggested that increased oxidative stress occurred in the nerve cells of transgenic Alzheimer's mice that were expressing mutated APP or presenilin-1.

Treatment of human neuroblastoma cells in culture with hydrogen peroxide (H_2O_2) significantly increased the production of beta-amyloids (Gu et al. 2013). This was due to the fact that increased oxidative stress elevated the activities of beta- and gamma-secretases responsible for the cleavage of APP to form beta-amyloids. These results suggest that increased oxidative stress enhanced the production of beta-amyloids.

Primary culture of neurons obtained from transgenic mice expressing both mutated APP and mutated presenilin-1 exhibited increased oxidative stress. It also increased sensitivity to oxidative damage induced by beta-amyloids, H_2O_2, and kainic acid. This contributed to the death of nerve cells (Mohmmad Abdul et al. 2006). These results also suggest that mutation in presenilin-1 and APP genes may cause neurodegeneration in patients with a family history of Alzheimer's disease via increasing oxidative stress.

Studies Utilizing Human Autopsied Brain Tissue

In a review it was shown that markers of oxidative stress (oxidized proteins, products of lipid oxidation, and oxidized DNA) were elevated in the autopsied samples of brains from patients with Alzheimer's (Sultana, Perluigi, and Butterfield 2006). A number of observations substantiate the presence of high levels of oxidative stress in patients with Alzheimer's disease. These results suggest that increased oxidative stress continues to occur and contribute to the progression of Alzheimer's.

Studies Utilizing Human Blood and Fibroblasts

The markers of oxidative stress were evaluated in peripheral tissue (blood and fibroblasts) to establish whether or not they can be used as a diagnostic tool to predict the presence of Alzheimer's disease and/

or mild cognitive impairment (MCI). The fibroblasts obtained from patients with a family history of Alzheimer's were more sensitive to oxidative stress than those obtained from age-matched, normal individuals (the controls) (Tesco et al. 1992).

The serum levels of vitamins A, E, and beta-carotene were lower in patients with Alzheimer's disease (who were well nourished) than in normal individuals (Zaman et al. 1992).

Increased levels of oxidized proteins were found in the blood of both Alzheimer's patients and their relatives when compared with controls not suffering from Alzheimer's (Conrad et al. 2000). This particular study reveals that increased oxidative stress occurs in the relatives of Alzheimer's disease patients who have no symptoms of the disease. This confirms the proposed hypothesis that increased oxidative stress is one of the earliest biochemical defects that initiate damage to the nerve cells in the brain of patients with Alzheimer's.

In a clinical study of eighty-two patients with Alzheimer's, forty-two with vascular dementia, and twenty-six healthy individuals, it was shown that the concentration of total serum antioxidant levels decreased, and the risk of medial temporal lobe atrophy (MTA) assessment increased in patients with Alzheimer's disease or vascular dementia (Zito et al. 2013).

In a clinical study of twelve patients with Alzheimer's disease, thirteen patients with non-Alzheimer's dementia, fourteen age-matched subjects, and fourteen young adult controls, it was demonstrated that elevated levels of markers of oxidative stress (H_2O_2 and organic hydroperoxides in red blood cells) were associated with age-related dementia, whereas decreased activity of glutathione peroxidase in red blood cells was associated with Alzheimer's (Kosenko et al. 2012). The authors suggested that the decreased activity of glutathione peroxidase in red blood cells can be used as a marker for Alzheimer's disease.

The results obtained on the serum levels of markers of oxidative stress in 101 patients with Alzheimer's disease and 134 patients with mild cognitive impairment suggested that increased levels of serum hydroperoxides were independently associated with the increased risk of developing mild cognitive impairment as well as Alzheimer's. However, low levels of serum total antioxidant capacity were associated with the increased risk of developing mild cognitive impairment (Cervellati et al. 2013).

In a clinical study of thirty-three patients with mild memory loss, twenty-nine patients with mild Alzheimer's, and twenty-six healthy age-matched subjects, it was demonstrated that plasma levels of malondialdehyde (MDA) were higher in patients with mild cognitive impairment and Alzheimer's disease than in control (normal healthy) subjects. Glutathione reductase activity in the red blood cells was lower in patients with mild cognitive impairment and Alzheimer's than in normal healthy subjects (Torres et al. 2011). These results suggest that increased oxidative stress is present in patients with an early stage of Alzheimer's disease.

In a clinical study of individuals carrying mutated preseniline-1 or mutated APP genes with no symptoms of Alzheimer's, and of their relatives who were not carrying a mutated gene, it was demonstrated that plasma markers of oxidative damage were elevated in individuals carrying a mutated gene with no symptoms of Alzheimer's disease in comparison to those in relatives with no mutated gene (Ringman et al. 2012). The results of this study provide the strongest support for the proposed hypothesis that increased oxidative stress is one of the earliest biochemical defects that initiate damage to the nerve cells in the brains of Alzheimer's patients.

Studies of Mitochondrial Defects

Most free radicals, as we have learned, are produced in the mitochondria. Mitochondria are very sensitive to free radical-induced damage in the adult nerve cells. One of the reasons could be that mitochondrial DNA (mtDNA) does not have genes to produce repair enzymes. Furthermore, unlike nuclear DNA, mtDNA is not shielded by protective histone proteins. mtDNA is present in close proximity to the site where free radicals are produced during the processing of oxygen to generate energy (Wallace 1992).

Such a location of mtDNA makes the mitochondria an easy target for free radicals. Indeed, an increased frequency of mutations in mtDNA has been found in the autopsy samples of the brains of people with Alzheimer's disease (Shoffner et al. 1993).

Several studies have implicated other types of mitochondrial defects in the development and progression of Alzheimer's (Mutisya, Bowling, and Beal 1994; Shoffner et al. 1993).

An increase in free Zn can impair mitochondrial function (Brown et al. 2000). An excess of free Zn is found in the autopsied brain samples of patients with Alzheimer's disease (Cuajungco and Lees 1998). Defective mitochondria produce more free radicals and less energy. This could then constitute a continuous cycle of the production of increased amounts of free radicals and enhanced mitochondrial dysfunction.

A review of several studies showed that some oxidized mitochondrial proteins were detected in the autopsied brain samples of Alzheimer's patients. In addition, decreased energy production was observed in patients with Alzheimer's disease exhibiting a mild cognitive dysfunction (Sultana and Butterfield 2009).

In another review it was shown that decreased energy production preceded the development of clinical symptoms of Alzheimer's disease (Piaceri et al. 2012).

Reduced brain energy production can also lead to hyperphosphorylation of tau protein and increased production of beta-amyloids. A study has reported that the peripheral lymphocytes obtained from patients with Alzheimer's, as well as from patients with mild cognitive impairment, exhibited mitochondrial dysfunction (Leuner et al. 2012).

Further studies revealed that Alzheimer's disease was associated with an early increase in markers of oxidative stress such as nitric oxide synthase and NADPH-oxidases, which could impair the mitochondrial function (de la Monte and Wands 2006). These studies reveal that mitochondrial dysfunction occurs in the early phase of Alzheimer's.

In a review it was shown that vascular and mitochondrial dysfunction and reduced energy production were commonly observed in patients with Alzheimer's disease. Vascular dysfunction included reduced blood flow to the brain and defects in the blood-brain barrier. These defects may reduce the clearance of beta-amyloids from the brain and thereby increase the deposits of beta-amyloids in the brain (Sochocka et al. 2013). Increased beta-amyloids contribute to the degeneration of nerve cells via free radicals.

Increased levels of reactive oxygen species induced chronic inflammation in the brain by increasing the expression and release of pro-inflammatory cytokines such as IL-1, IL-6, TNF-alpha, and chemokines that are toxic to nerve cells. Chronic inflammation then activates microglia and astrocytes, which further enhances the levels of reactive oxygen species. Hence, chronic inflammation may serve as a constant source of free radicals. Increased oxidative stress can lead to enhanced production of beta-amyloids in the brain that are toxic to the nerve cells.

The results discussed in the paragraphs above suggest that increased oxidative stress is one of the earliest biochemical defects initiating mitochondrial dysfunction, inducing chronic inflammation, and increasing production of beta-amyloids, all of which participate in the progression of Alzheimer's disease.

Studies Involving Beta-Amyloids

Increased production and aggregation of beta-amyloids contribute to the death of nerve cells in the brains of patients with Alzheimer's. It is now established that beta-amyloids, also called Aß-1-42 peptides, are produced by cleavage of the amyloid precursor protein (APP) by the enzymes beta- and gamma-secretase, which play a central role in the development and progression of Alzheimer's disease (Selkoe 1994; Yankner and Mesulam 1991).

Increased oxidative stress may enhance production and accumulation of beta-amyloids in the nerve cells (Misonou, Morishima-Kawashima, and Ihara 2000). This was confirmed in a transgenic Alzheimer's mouse model lacking cytoplasmic superoxide dismutase-1 (SOD-1). Lack of SOD-1 would increase oxidative stress in these mice. This study demonstrated that the rate of cleavage of APP to beta-amyloids was elevated due to increased oxidative stress in transgenic mice compared to mice that contained SOD-1. These results suggested that an increase in oxidative stress in the nerve cells can increase the production of beta-amyloids (Murakami et al. 2012).

It has been shown that aggregates of beta-amyloids are toxic to neurons in culture (Schubert et al. 1995; Lorenzo and Yankner 1994). Several agents can enhance the aggregation of beta-amyloids. They include excess amounts of free Zn and Cu (Koh et al. 1996), iron, and aluminum (Bondy and Truong 1999), and complement proteins (Eikelenboom and Stam 1982).

It was further demonstrated that iron enhances beta-amyloid toxicity (Liu et al. 2011). The role of iron-beta-amyloid complexes in the development and progression of Alzheimer's disease is supported by the fact that the administration of iron increased the levels of APP and the production and deposition of beta-amyloids and impaired learning ability and memory in the transgenic mouse Alzheimer's model. Administration of deferoxamine, a chelator of iron, prevented the damaging effects of iron on the nerve cells (Guo, Wang, Zheng, et al. 2013).

Curcumin, derived from turmeric, which exhibits antioxidant and anti-inflammatory activities, binds with iron and copper more readily than with zinc. Therefore, curcumin treatment may prevent iron- and copper-induced aggregation of beta-amyloids, their deposition, and toxicity (Baum and Ng 2004).

Beta-amyloid aggregates are insoluble; however, soluble beta-amyloid-oligomer, which contains an aggregation of fewer than four identical beta-amyloids, is also formed. Beta-amyloid oligomers trigger increased levels of oxidative stress, which induces inflammation. This is evidenced by the presence on an increased number of astrocytes in the brains of patients with Alzheimer's disease (Alberdi et al. 2013).

In mature hippocampal neurons in culture, it was demonstrated that beta-amyloid oligomers caused disassembly of microtubules and induced DNA fragmentation within the nerve cells. Beta-amyloids may also contribute to the degeneration of synapses that connect the nerve cells (Mota et al. 2012).

The aggregated form of beta-amyloid participates in the formation of senile plaque. This can serve as a chronic source of inflammatory reactions, the products of which can enhance the progressive degeneration of nerve cells.

Studies Involving the Impacts of Free Radicals on Beta-Amyloids

It has been proposed that one of the mechanisms of action of beta-amyloid-induced neurotoxicity (damage in the nerve cells) is mediated by free radicals (Schubert et al. 1995; Butterfield et al. 1994; Behl et al. 1994).

This is supported by the fact that vitamin E protects nerve cells in culture against beta-amyloid-induced toxicity (Behl et al. 1992). Binding of beta-amyloid with red blood cells impairs delivery of oxygen to the brain tissue, which increases oxidative stress. The binding of copper with beta-amyloid (copper-beta-amyloid complex) caused the formation of aggregates that produce excessive amounts of free radicals, which caused an increased oxidation of hemoglobin (damage to hemoglobin by free radicals) (Lucas and Rifkind 2013).

These data suggest that the copper-beta-amyloid complex damages blood vessels via free radicals. Damaged blood vessels reduce oxygen delivery to the brain, resulting in degeneration and, eventually, death of the nerve cells.

Studies Involving the Cholesterol-Induced Production of Beta-Amyloids

Epidemiologic (survey-type) studies have found that hypercholesterolemia (very high levels of cholesterol in the blood) may increase the risk of developing Alzheimer's disease (Wolozin et al. 2000; Sparks et al. 2000).

This was confirmed in the transgenic animal model of Alzheimer's (Sparks et al. 2000). Another study revealed that high dietary cholesterol increased the accumulation of beta-amyloids and accelerated neurodegenerative changes in the brain of transgenic Alzheimer's animals (Refolo et al. 2000).

The accumulation of beta-amyloids can be reversed by removing cholesterol from the animal's diet. The enzyme HMG CoA reductase (3-hydroxy-3-methyl-glutaryl-CoA reductase) is responsible for the formation of cholesterol. Inhibitors of HMG CoA reductase activity, such as statin, decrease production of beta-amyloids in rabbits (Sparks et al. 2000).

An epidemiologic study has shown that lovastatin, an inhibitor of HMG CoA reductase, reduced the risk of Alzheimer's disease in hypercholesterolemic patients (Jick et al. 2000).

In another epidemiologic study the use of statins, but not of nonstatin cholesterol-lowering drugs, was associated with a reduced incidence of Alzheimer's in comparison to those who had never taken statins (Haag et al. 2009).

These results suggest that lower levels of cholesterol may reduce the risk of developing Alzheimer's. High cholesterol levels may increase the risk of developing Alzheimer's disease by producing increased amounts of beta-amyloids, which causes degeneration of the nerve cells via an increased production of free radicals.

Studies Revealing That Mutated Genes Increase Production of Beta-Amyloids in Familial Alzheimer's Disease

In some cases of familial Alzheimer's disease, mutations (about seven) in the APP gene have been reported, all of which increase the production of beta-amyloids (Sherrington et al. 1995). However, this accounts for less than 1 percent of all familial Alzheimer's cases.

Mutations (about fifty) in presenilin-1 gene have been found in about 50 percent of familial Alzheimer's disease (Sherrington et al. 1995), whereas mutations in presenilin-2 gene have been observed in less than 1 percent of familial Alzheimer's. Presenilin-1 protein is present in senile plaques and NTFs of Alzheimer's brains (Sherrington et al. 1995).

Mutations in APP and presenilin-1 genes increase the production of beta-amyloids by increasing gamma-secretase activity (Tabaton and Tamagno 2007). Increased beta-amyloids cause death of the nerve cells by increasing oxidative stress in primary cultures of brain nerve cells in mice (Mohmmad Abdul et al. 2006). The levels of oxidative damage as a function of age were more pronounced in mice expressing mutant human APP and presenilin-1 genes in comparison with those observed in normal mice (Abdul et al. 2008).

Mutation in the gamma-secretase gene causes a rare form of early onset Alzheimer's disease due to the production of increased amounts of beta-amyloids (Placanica et al. 2009). The activity of gamma-secretase increases as a function of age in female mice (Placanica et al. 2009). This may, in part, be responsible for the relatively increased incidence of Alzheimer's in women.

These studies suggest that mutations in both APP and presenilin-1 increase the rate of production of beta-amyloids. Excessive production of beta-amyloids can generate more free radicals, inhibit proteasome activity, and contribute to the formation of senile plaques, all of which contribute to the progressive loss of nerve cells in the brain of the person with Alzheimer's disease.

Studies Measuring the Markers of Chronic Inflammation in Alzheimer's Disease

Evidence of the presence of chronic inflammation in autopsied brain tissue from patients with Alzheimer's disease was first observed by Dr. Alois Alzheimer himself. The role of chronic inflammation in the development and progression of Alzheimer's disease is supported by the epidemiologic (survey-type) studies that showed that rheumatoid arthritis patients who were on high doses of nonsteroidal anti-inflammatory agents (NSAIDs) had a reduced incidence of Alzheimer's (McGeer and McGeer 1998).

Direct evidence supporting the role of chronic inflammation in the degeneration of nerve cells came from laboratory experiments in which the products of chronic inflammatory reaction such as cytokines (Shalit et al. 1994), complement proteins (Rogers et al. 1995; Webster et al. 1994), free radicals (Chen et al. 1994; Smith et al. 1995; Harman 1992), adhesion molecules (Frohman et al. 1991; Verbeek et al. 1994), and prostaglandins (Prasad et al. 1998) produced degeneration and death of the nerve cells.

Increased levels of pro-inflammatory cytokines such as IL-1 beta and TNF-alpha were found in the autopsied brain tissue of Alzheimer's patients (Sutton et al. 1999).

Beta-amyloids also caused a disruption of blood vessel function in the Alzheimer's brain, which is mediated through the pro-inflammatory cytokines TNF-alpha and IL-1 beta (Ramirez, Rey, and von Bernhardi 2008; Yamamoto et al. 2007).

Beta-amyloid-induced toxicity in the nerve cells can be enhanced by the pro-inflammatory cytokines IL-1beta and TNF-alpha (Ramirez, Rey, and von Bernhardi 2008). The pro-inflammatory cytokines interferon-gamma, IL-1beta, and TNF-alpha increased the activity of gamma-secretase, which enhanced the production of beta-amyloids from APP (Liao et al. 2004). The cycle of increased chronic inflammation causing increased production of beta-amyloids, which then induce chronic inflammation, is repeated during the progression of Alzheimer's disease. This results in increased oxidative stress and death of the nerve cells.

The role of inflammatory reactions in the development and progression of Alzheimer's was further supported by clinical studies in which the administration of NSAIDs reduced the rate of deterioration of cognitive function in moderate to advanced Alzheimer's patients (Rich et al. 1995; Lucca et al. 1994; Rogers et al. 1993).

However, clinical studies with two new NSAIDs (celecoxib and naproxen) on men and women aged seventy years or more with a familial history of Alzheimer's disease revealed that these drugs did not improve cognitive function. On the contrary detrimental effects of naproxen were observed in some patients with Alzheimer's (Martin et al. 2008).

It has been reported that NSAIDs such as ibuprofen, aspirin, indomethacin, and naproxen inhibited to a varying degree formation of beta-amyloid aggregates and destabilized preformed beta-amyloid aggregates in vitro (Hirohata et al. 2005).

Ibuprofen reduced the levels of beta-amyloids and hyperphosphorylated tau protein and improved memory deficits in Alzheimer's transgenic mice (McKee et al. 2008).

These studies suggest that chronic inflammation plays an important role in the development and progression of Alzheimer's disease.

Studies Pertaining to the Role of Hyperphosphorylated and Acetylated Tau Protein in Alzheimer's Disease

Tau is a microtubule-binding protein and a major component of neurofibrillary tangles that are present inside the nerve cells of the brain of an Alzheimer's patient. Increased oxidative stress causes hyperphosphorylation of tau protein (P-tau) in transgenic Alzheimer's disease model of mice (Tg2576). This hyperphosphorylation of tau protein was prevented by high doses of antioxidants (Melov et al. 2007), confirming the role of oxidative stress in the hyperphosphorylation of tau protein.

It has been shown that an increase in beta-amyloids precedes the hyperphosphorylation of tau protein and the formation of neurofibrillary tangles in the cortex region of the brain (Naslund et al. 2000). Tau protein is present in axons as well as at presynaptic and postsynaptic terminals in the normal human brain. However, in the Alzheimer's brain tau becomes hyperphosphorylated and misfolded at both pre- and postsynaptic terminals.

The accumulation of hyperphosphorylated tau protein oligomers at the synapses inhibited proteasome activity and disrupted synaptic function (Tai et al. 2012). Hyperphosphorylated tau protein in aggregated and oligomer forms disrupts microtubules, causing loss of connectivity between the nerve cells (Iqbal et al. 2009).

The activity of protein phosphatase-2A (PP-2A) is decreased in the Alzheimer's brain, causing hyperphosphorylation of tau. Zinc is widely distributed in the brain but accumulated in the Alzheimer's disease affected areas of the brain more than in other areas. It has been reported that zinc caused the hyperphosphorylation of tau by inhibiting PP-2A activity in the rat brain (Xiong et al. 2013). Chelation of zinc completely prevented zinc-induced hyperphosphorylation of tau protein.

In addition to hyperphosphorylation of tau protein, acetylation of tau protein occurs in the Alzheimer's brain. Acetylated tau protein is present within the neuron of the hippocampus of patients with Alzheimer's disease. The distribution pattern of acetylated tau protein is similar to that of P-tau protein, and it is present in all stages of the disease. However, it is markedly elevated at the advanced stage of the disease when the levels of hyperphosphorylated tau protein are also elevated (Irwin et al. 2012). Thus, it appears that the acetylation of tau protein also participates in the progression of Alzheimer's disease.

Studies Pertaining to the Role of Proteasome Inhibition-Induced Neurodegeneration in Alzheimer's Disease

One of the functions of proteasome is to remove abnormal proteins, because if they're allowed to accumulate, they may cause the death of nerve cells. Inhibition of proteasome activity can therefore cause the degeneration and death of nerve cells. Indeed, the role of proteasome inhibition has been proposed for the degeneration of neurons in Alzheimer's brains (Gregori et al. 1997; Checler et al. 2000).

In our study inhibition of proteasome activity by lactacystin caused the rapid degeneration of nerve cells in culture (Nahreini, Andreatta, and Prasad 2001). Several factors can inhibit proteasome activity. They include increased oxidative stress, defects in ubiquitin conjugate enzymes (Lopez Salon et al. 2000), mutations in ubiquitin (Lam et al. 2000), and excess levels of beta-amyloids (Gregori et al. 1997). The exact mechanisms of proteasome inhibition in the Alzheimer's disease neurons are unknown, but increased oxidative stress may be one of the earliest biochemical defects that can inhibit proteasome activity.

Studies Pertaining to the Role of Apolipoprotein (APOE) in Alzheimer's Disease

Apolipoprotein E (APOE) is present in the high-density lipoprotein-like particles in the brain and appears to be involved in various protective anti-inflammatory and antioxidant functions as well as in cholesterol transport. Administration of an APOE mimetic peptide (Ac-hE18A-NH2) in transgenic Alzheimer's mice (human APP/PS1ΔE9) for a period of six weeks improved cognitive function, reduced amyloid plaque deposition, and reduced activated microglia and astrocytes. APOE mimetic peptide also reduced oxidative-stress-induced APOE secretion (Handattu et al. 2013). These results suggest that high levels of APOE in the brain could reduce the development of Alzheimer's disease.

Several studies have suggested that persons who are homozygous for the APOE4 allele develop Alzheimer's disease ten to twenty years earlier than those who have APOE2 allele or APOE3 allele (Farrer et al. 1997; Marx 1998).

Even persons who are heterozygous for APOE4 allele develop Alzheimer's five to ten years earlier than those who have APOE2 allele or APOE3 allele (McConnell et al. 1998). About 40 percent of Alzheimer's cases are associated with the presence of APOE4 allele (McConnell et al. 1998).

These data suggest that the presence of APOE4 allele could be an important risk factor for the development Alzheimer's disease. The results of a clinical study showed that an annual increase in the levels of F2-isoprostanes (a marker of oxidative stress) was greater in patients carrying APOE4 allele than in patients who carry no ApoE4 allele. An increase in F2-isoprostane levels was associated with enhanced cognitive dysfunction in patients with APOE4 allele compared to patients who did not carry APOE4 allele.

These studies further suggest the presence of increased oxidative stress in patients carrying APOE4 allele, indicating that this genetic defect participates in the development and progression of Alzheimer's disease (Duits et al. 2013).

APOE4 allele also stimulated the accumulation of beta-amyloids and hyperphosphorylated tau protein and caused cognitive dysfunction (Liraz, Boehm-Cagan, and Michaelson 2013).

Studies Pertaining to the Role of a Nuclear Transcriptional Factor-2 (Nrf2) in Alzheimer's Disease

The Nrf2 is a transcriptional factor that regulates antioxidant genes responsible for producing antioxidant enzymes in the nerve cells. Nrf2 is present in both the cytoplasm and the nucleus of the nerve cells. Normally, in response to increased oxidative stress, Nrf2 is activated and translocates itself from the cytoplasm to the nucleus where it binds with ARE (antioxidant response elements) to enhance the expression of antioxidant genes responsible for producing antioxidant enzymes.

The levels of Nrf2 were decreased in the brains of Alzheimer's patients (Ramsey et al. 2007).

In addition, activation of Nrf2 becomes unresponsive to increased oxidative stress. These results suggest that one of the brain's normal protective responses against free radical damage becomes impaired in Alzheimer's disease. It's possible that increased chronic oxidative stress overwhelms this normal neuroprotective response.

These data suggest that activation of Nrf2 may reduce the development and progression of Alzheimer's. Indeed, treatment with tert-butylhydroquinone, a known inducer of Nrf2, protected neurons against beta-amyloid-induced damage to the nerve cells in transgenic Alzheimer's mice (Kanninen et al. 2008).

CONCLUDING REMARKS

Despite extensive laboratory and clinical studies, it has not been possible to reduce the incidence or the rate of progression of Alzheimer's although the scientific community has been able to identify several internal and external risk factors that are implicated in the onset and progression of the disease.

Coupled with this are the extensive research studies that have been done, which attempt to determine the causative factors of the disease. Biochemical and genetic defects have been identified by these studies. In the brains of people with Alzheimer's, these defects are deemed to be responsible for the death of neurons in the brain. Increased oxidative stress together with other biochemical and genetic defects helps to accelerate the disease.

Activation of nuclear transcriptional factor-2 (Nrf2) reduces oxidative stress indirectly by increasing the levels of antioxidant enzymes. Antioxidants present in the body reduce oxidative stress by directly scavenging free radicals. When oxidative stress occurs Nrf2 is activated and translocates itself from the cytoplasm of the cell to its nucleus. Here, via the antioxidant response elements, it enhances the expression of antioxidant genes responsible for making antioxidant enzymes.

Certain studies have found that the levels of Nrf2 were decreased in the brains of Alzheimer's patients. It is also true that the activation of Nrf2 becomes impaired despite elevated levels of oxidative stress. These results suggest that one of the brain's normal protective responses against free radical damage becomes damaged in the case of Alzheimer's disease.

Given that antioxidants may be our best hope in combatting Alzheimer's disease, let's look at them next. In chapter 4 we will profile many different types of antioxidants. In so doing we will discuss the various characteristics and properties of these very beneficial substances.

4 The Antioxidant Defense System

This chapter presents a broad overview of antioxidants and as such details many of their qualities and characteristics. This discussion is important for a more enhanced understanding of these valuable substances and will be a useful guide for those individuals seeking a greater inclusion of them through diet or supplementation. Specifically, the discussion in this chapter centers around the history, functions, sources and forms, absorption, solubility, and availability of antioxidants. It also covers other practical matters such as how to most effectively store antioxidants in the home and whether or not they may be destroyed in cooking.

It's vital to have this full complement of knowledge about antioxidants so that we may more completely grasp the ensuing discussion in chapter 5. That discussion examines how, specifically, antioxidants help the body fight increased oxidative stress and inflammation, thereby helping to prevent and mitigate the debilitating effects of Alzheimer's disease.

A CLOSER LOOK AT ANTIOXIDANTS

Antioxidants are chemical micronutrients that donate an electron to a free radical and convert it into a harmless molecule. They are considered to be micronutrients. But what exactly is a micronutrient? In defining micronutrients it's important to distinguish them from macronutrients. Primarily, macronutrients include fats, carbohydrates, and proteins. Micronutrients, on the other hand, include antioxidant systems represented by dietary and endogenous (made in the body) antioxidant chemicals; polyphenolic compounds derived from fruits, vegetables, and plants; the mineral selenium; and B vitamins as well as vitamin D. Antioxidant enzymes represent one of the components of the antioxidant system; other components include dietary and endogenous antioxidant chemicals.

Although *all* micronutrients are essential for human survival and growth, antioxidants have enjoyed a special focus in this regard. They have been the subject of extensive laboratory research and clinical studies because of their potential importance in reducing oxidative stress and inflammation, which could decrease the risk of chronic disease.

Polyphenolic compounds derived from herbs also exhibit antioxidant and anti-inflammatory activities; however, they act in part by different mechanisms. Some of them reduce oxidative stress by activating the nuclear transcription factor Nrf2, which increases the levels of antioxidant enzymes by upregulating the antioxidant genes through antioxidant response elements. Some dietary and endogenous antioxidants also activate Nrf2 by a ROS-independent mechanism. Therefore, a combination of antioxidant chemicals and polyphenolic compounds may reduce oxidative stress and inflammation optimally.

The antioxidant defense system in humans can be divided into four groups, which we will look at next.

Group 1 Antioxidants

These antioxidants are not made in the body but are consumed primarily through the diet. They include vitamin A, carotenoids, vitamin C, vitamin E, and selenium. They scavenge free radicals directly.

Group 2 Antioxidants

Group 2 antioxidants are made in the body and are also consumed through the diet (primarily through meat and eggs) or in the form of supplements. They include glutathione, coenzyme Q10, α-lipoic acid, and L-carnitine.

Group 3 Antioxidants

Group 3 antioxidants include antioxidants derived from fruit, vegetables, and plants. They also include polyphenolic compounds such as curcumin and resveratrol, which can be taken through the diet. However, dietary sources of these polyphenolic compounds may not provide sufficient amounts needed for the prevention of chronic neurological diseases. Thus, supplementation may be necessary for optimal biological activity in the body. Both curcumin and resveratrol activate a nuclear transcriptional factor, Nrf2, which increases the levels of antioxidant enzymes by upregulating the expression of antioxidant genes through the antioxidant response elements.

Group 4 Antioxidants

Another form of antioxidants are antioxidant enzymes that are made in the body. They include superoxide dismutase (SOD), catalase, and glutathione peroxidase, all of which destroy free radicals by catalysis (converting free radicals to harmless chemicals). Superoxide dismutase requires manganese (Mn) or copper (Cu)-zinc SOD for its biological activity. Mn-SOD is present in the mitochondria, whereas Cu-Zn SOD is present in the cytoplasm. Both can destroy free radicals and hydrogen peroxide. Catalase requires iron (Fe) for its biological activity. It, too, destroys hydrogen peroxide in the cell. Glutathione peroxidase requires selenium for its biological activity.

THE ROLE OF ANTIOXIDANTS

Antioxidants have many valuable roles to play in safeguarding human health. Given that they're so successful in neutralizing free radicals, many people believe that this is their only function. However, in view of recent advances in antioxidant research, this belief has been proven to be incorrect. The actions of antioxidants on cells and tissues are varied and complex. Antioxidants and polyphenolic compounds work to:

1. Scavenge free radicals
2. Decrease markers of pro-inflammatory cytokines
3. Alter gene expression profiles
4. Alter protein kinase activity
5. Prevent the release and toxicity of excessive amounts of glutamate
6. Act as cofactors for several biological reactions
7. Induce cell differentiation and apoptosis in cancer cells
8. Induce cell differentiation in normal cells, but not apoptosis
9. Increase immune function
10. Activate a nuclear transcriptional factor Nrf2 that translocates itself from the cytoplasm to the nucleus

HISTORY OF ANTIOXIDANTS

Vitamin A

Night blindness existed for centuries before the discovery of vitamin A. As early as 1500 BCE Egyptians knew how to cure night blindness. Roman soldiers suffering from this condition traveled to Egypt where they received liver extract as treatment. (Today it is well established that liver is the richest source of vitamin A.) Treating night blindness with liver extract was not employed outside of Egypt for centuries, perhaps because medical establishments in other countries during that time period did not deem it to be an acceptable treatment protocol.

In 1912 Dr. Elmer McCollum of the University of Wisconsin discovered vitamin A in butter, at which time it was named "fat-soluble A." The structure of vitamin A was determined in 1930, and it was synthesized in the laboratory in 1947.

It should be underscored that the medical establishment of that very early period, by denying the validity of vitamin A to cure night blindness, no doubt delayed the cure for blindness for centuries.

The Vitamin B Family

All of the B vitamins were discovered between 1912 and 1934. In the year 1912 the Polish biochemist Dr. Casimur Funk isolated their active substances from the rice husks of unpolished rice; these active substances prevented the disease beriberi. This disease affects many parts of the body including muscle tissue, the heart, the nervous system, and the digestive tract. Dr. Funk named the substances he discovered vitamines, because he thought they were "amines" derived from ammonia. In 1920 the e was dropped when it became known that not all vitamins are "amines." Today there are many different vitamins in the vitamin B family.

Vitamin C

Vitamin C deficiency causes scurvy, the symptoms of which were known to Egyptians as early as 1500 BCE. In the fifth century Hippocrates described these symptoms. They include bleeding gums, hemorrhaging, and death. Native Americans had a cure for scurvy, which involved drinking an extract made from the bark and needles of the pine tree, prepared like a tea. This remedy, however, remained limited to their own population for hundreds of years. Today we know that pine bark and needles are rich in vitamin C.

During the sea voyages of European explorers between the twelfth and sixteenth centuries, the epidemic of scurvy among sailors forced some of them to land in Canada, where native Indians gave them the indigenous concoction, thereby curing their illness. In 1536 the French explorer Jacques Cartier brought this formulation to France, but the medical establishment rejected it as bogus because it had originated with the Native Americans, whom they looked down upon. In 1593 Sir Richard Hawkins began recommending that his sailors eat sour oranges and lemons to reduce the risk of disease. It would be almost another two hundred years before the British Navy began recommending that ships carry sufficient lime juice for all personnel aboard. In 1928 Albert Szent-Györgyi, a Hungarian scientist, isolated hexuronic acid from the adrenal gland. This substance was vitamin C, and in 1932 it was the first vitamin to be made in the laboratory.

It should be emphasized that the sixteenth-century medical community in France, by rejecting the use of vitamin C to treat scurvy, delayed the cure of this disease for centuries.

Carotenoids/Beta-Carotene
In 1919 carotenoid pigments were isolated from yellow plants, and in 1930 researchers found that some of the ingested carotene was converted to vitamin A. This substance is referred to as beta-carotene.

Vitamin D
Although the bone disease rickets may have existed in human populations for a long time, it wasn't until 1645 that Dr. Daniel Whistler described its symptoms. In 1922 Sir Edward Mellanby discovered vitamin D while working on a cure for rickets, which vitamin D proved to be. This vitamin was later found to require sunlight for its formation in the skin cells. The chemical structure of vitamin D was determined by German scientist Dr. Adolf Windaus in 1930. Vitamin D_3 is the most active form of vitamin D. It was chemically characterized in 1936 and was initially thought to be a steroid effective in the treatment of rickets.

Vitamin E

In 1922 Dr. Herbert Evans of the University of California, Berkeley, observed that rats reared exclusively on whole milk grew normally but were not fertile. Fertility was restored when they were fed wheat germ. However, it took another fourteen years before the active substance that was responsible for restoring fertility was isolated. When this was achieved, Dr. Evans named the substance tocopherol, from the Greek word meaning "to bear offspring" and then added *ol* to the end, signifying its chemical status as an alcohol.

Coenzyme Q10

In 1957 Dr. Fredrick Crane isolated coenzyme Q10. In 1958 Dr. Wolf, working under Dr. Karl Folkers, determined the structure of coenzyme Q10.

FUNCTIONS
OF SPECIFIC ANTIOXIDANTS

Vitamin A

In addition to destroying free radicals, vitamin A plays an important role in maintaining vision and skin health; stimulating immune function; in bone metabolism; regulating gene activity, embryonic development, and reproduction; and inhibiting precancerous and cancerous cell proliferation.

Alpha-Lipoic Acid

Alpha-lipoic acid is a more potent antioxidant than vitamin C or vitamin E. It's soluble in both water and lipid and thus protects cellular membranes as well as water-soluble compounds. It regenerates tissue levels of vitamin C and vitamin E and markedly elevates glutathione levels in the cells. Alpha-lipoic acid acts as a cofactor for multienzyme dehydrogenase complexes.

Vitamin C

Vitamin C acts as an antioxidant and participates as a cofactor for the activities of some enzymes, which is essential for the formation of many vital compounds in our body. Vitamin C helps in the formation of collagen, and it also takes part in the formation of interferon, a naturally occurring antiviral agent. It regenerates oxidized vitamin E to a reduced form, which acts as an antioxidant.

Carotenoids

Beta-carotene is a precursor of vitamin A. Carotenes are known to protect against ultraviolet-light-induced damage. Beta-carotene increases the expression of the connexin gene, which codes for a gap junction protein that holds two normal cells together. (Vitamin A can't produce such an effect.) In addition, when compared to vitamins A and E, beta-carotene is a more effective destroyer of free radicals in an internal body environment that is marked by high oxygen pressure in the tissues.

Coenzyme Q10

Coenzyme Q10 is a weak antioxidant, but it recycles oxidized vitamin E to a reduced form that acts as an antioxidant. Coenzyme Q10 is essential in generating energy by the mitochondria.

Vitamin D$_3$

Vitamin D$_3$ is essential for bone formation, and regulates calcium and phosphorus levels in the blood. Vitamin D$_3$ also inhibits parathyroid hormone secretion from the parathyroid glands. It stimulates immune function by promoting phagocytosis and also exhibits antitumor activity.

Vitamin E

Vitamin E acts as an antioxidant and regulates gene expression. It also translocates certain proteins from one cellular compartment to another. Additionally, it helps to maintain skin texture, reduces scarring, and acts as an anticoagulant. Vitamin E reduces inflammation and stimulates immune function. Its derivative, vitamin E succinate, exhibits potent anticancer activities.

Glutathione

Glutathione is one of the most important antioxidants in that it protects cellular components inside the cells. It is needed for the detoxification of toxins, either certain exogenous toxins or those generated as by-products of normal metabolism. Glutathione also acts as a substrate for several enzymes. It reduces inflammation.

Melatonin

Melatonin is important in regulating circadian rhythms through its receptor. It also acts as an antioxidant and reduces inflammation. Unlike other antioxidants, the oxidation of melatonin is irreversible and thus cannot be regenerated by other antioxidants. Melatonin also stimulates immune function.

N-acetylcysteine (NAC)

N-acetylcysteine increases the glutathione levels within the cells. This function is important because orally administered glutathione is totally destroyed in the small intestine. At high doses N-acetylcysteine binds with metals and removes them from the body.

Nicotinamide (Vitamin B_3)

Treatment with nicotinamide restored memory deficits in Alzheimer's disease transgenic mice (Green et al. 2008), attenuated glutamate-induced toxicity, and preserved cellular levels of NAD+ to support the activity of SIRT-1 (Liu, Pitta, and Mattson 2008). Treatment with nicotinamide reduced oxidative-stress-induced mitochondrial dysfunction and increased the survival of neurons in culture. The reduced form of NAD (NADH) acts as an antioxidant and is essential for generating energy by the mitochondria.

Polyphenolic Compounds

Polyphenolic compounds exhibit antioxidant activity and reduce inflammation. They also regulate the expression of certain genes. Some polyphenolic compounds such as resveratrol and curcumin also increase the levels of antioxidant enzymes by activating a nuclear transcriptional factor, Nrf2.

SOURCES AND FORMS OF ANTIOXIDANTS

Vitamin A

Liver from beef, pork, chicken, turkey, and fish is the richest source of vitamin A (6.5 milligrams per 100 grams of liver). Other rich sources are carrot (0.8 milligrams per 100 grams), broccoli (0.8 milligrams per 100 grams), sweet potato (0.7 milligrams per 100 grams), kale (0.7 milligrams per 100 grams), butter (0.7 milligrams per 100 grams), spinach (0.5 milligrams per 100 grams), and pumpkin (0.4 milligrams per 100 grams). Minor sources include cantaloupe melon, egg, apricot, papaya, and mango (40 to 170 micrograms per 100 grams). Yellow and red fruits and vegetables are very rich sources of beta-carotene. One molecule of beta-carotene is converted to two molecules of retinol (vitamin A) in the intestinal tract.

Vitamin A exists as retinyl palmitate or retinyl acetate that's converted into the retinol form in the body. Vitamin A exists as a retinoic acid in the cells. It has been determined that 1 IU (international unit) equals 0.3 micrograms of retinol or 0.6 micrograms of beta-carotene. The activity of vitamin A is also expressed as retinol activity equivalent (RAE). One microgram of RAE corresponds to 1 microgram of retinol and 2 micrograms of beta-carotene in oil. Vitamin A, beta-carotene, and the synthetic retinoids are also available commercially.

Vitamin C

The richest source of vitamin C is fruits and vegetables, which include rose hip (2,000 milligrams per 100 grams of rose hip), red pepper (2,000 milligrams per 100 grams of red pepper), parsley (2,000 milligrams per 100 grams of parsley), guava (2,000 milligrams per 100 grams of guava), kiwi fruit (2,000 milligrams per 100 grams of kiwi fruit), broccoli (2,000 milligrams per 100 grams of broccoli), lychee (2,000 milligrams per 100 grams of lychee), papaya (2,000 milligrams per 100 grams of papaya), and strawberry (2,000 milligrams per 100 grams of strawberry). Other sources of vitamin C include orange, lemon, melon, garlic, cauliflower, grapefruit, raspberry, tangerine, passion fruit, spinach, and lime. These foods contain about 30 to 50 milligrams per 100 grams of fruits and vegetables. Vitamin C is sold commercially as L-ascorbic acid, calcium ascorbate, sodium ascorbate, and potassium ascorbate.

Carotenoids

The richest sources of carotenoids are sweet potato, carrot, spinach, mango, cantaloupe, apricot, kale, broccoli, parsley, cilantro, pumpkin, winter squash, and fresh thyme. There are two main forms of carotenoids found in nature: alpha-carotene and beta-carotene. Beta-carotene is one of the more than 600 carotenoids found in fruits, vegetables, and plants and represents the more common form of carotenoids. Other carotenes include lutein and lycopene.

Vitamin E

The richest sources of vitamin E include wheat germ oil (215 milligrams per 100 grams of oil), sunflower oil (56 milligrams per 100 grams of oil), olive oil (12 milligrams per 100 grams of oil), almond oil (39 milligrams per 100 grams of oil), hazelnut oil (26 milligrams per 100 grams of oil), walnut oil (20 milligrams per 100 grams of oil), and peanut oil (17 milligrams per 100 grams of oil). The sources for small amounts of vitamin E (0.1 to 2 milligrams per 100 grams) include kiwi fruit, fish, leafy vegetables, and whole grains. In the United States fortified breakfast cereal is an important source of vitamin E. At present the natural form of vitamin E is primarily extracted from vegetable oil, particularly soybean oil.

Vitamin E exists in eight different forms: four tocopherols (alpha-, beta-, gamma-, and delta-tocopherol) and four tocotrienols (alpha-, beta-, gamma-, and delta-tocotrienol). Alpha-tocopherol has the most biological activity. Vitamin E exists in the natural form commonly indicated as "d," whereas the synthetic form is referred to as "dl." The stable esterified form of vitamin E is available as alpha-tocopheryl acetate, alpha-tocopheryl succinate, and alpha-tocopheryl nicotinate. The activity of vitamin E is generally expressed in international units (IU). It is determined that 1 IU equals 0.66 milligrams of d-alpha-tocopherol, and 1 IU of racemic mixture (dl-form) equals 0.45 milligrams of d-tocopherol.

Glutathione

Glutathione is synthesized from three amino acids: L-cysteine, L-glutamic acid, and L-glycine, and is present in all cells of the body. However, its highest concentration is found in the liver. Glutathione exists in the cells in a reduced or oxidized form. In healthy cells more than 90 percent of glutathione is present in the reduced form. The oxidized form of glutathione can be converted to the reduced form by the enzyme glutathione reductase. The reduced form of glutathione acts as an antioxidant.

L-carnitine

L-carnitine was originally found to be a growth factor for mealworms. It is synthesized, primarily in the liver and kidney, from the amino acids lysine and methionine. Vitamin C is necessary for its synthesis. It exists as R-L-carnitine, a biologically active form, and as D-carnitine, a biologically inactive form.

Polyphenolic Compounds

Polyphenolic compounds are found in herbs, fruits, vegetables, and plants. They include tannins, lignins, and flavonoids. The most widely studied polyphenolic compounds are flavonoids, which include resveratrol (in grape skin and seed), curcumin (in spices such as turmeric), ginseng extract, cinnamon extract, garlic extract, quercetin, epicatechin, and oligomeric proanthocyanidins. Major sources of flavonoids include all citrus fruit, berries, ginkgo biloba, onion, parsley, tea, red wine, and dark chocolate. Over five thousand naturally occurring flavonoids have been characterized from various plants.

ABSORPTION OF ANTIOXIDANTS

Antioxidants are absorbed from the intestinal tract and then distributed to various organs of the body. The highest levels of vitamin A, C, and E are present in the liver, and the lowest levels of these antioxidants are in the brain. Regarding coenzyme Q10 the heart and the liver have the highest levels of it. Only about 10 percent of ingested water-soluble and fat-soluble antioxidants are absorbed from the intestinal tract. It has been argued by some that 90 percent of antioxidants are therefore wasted but this argument has no scientific merit.

During the process of digestion, many toxic substances including mutagens (agents that can alter genetic activity) and carcinogens (agents that can cause cancer) are formed. What's interesting to note is that the consumption of organic food makes little difference in the amount of toxins formed during the digestive process. Organic food may, however, be devoid of pesticides, although these pesticides represent only about 1 percent of naturally occurring toxins. Pesticides are not metabolized and are difficult to remove from the body.

The formation of toxins is more prevalent in meat eaters than in vegetarians. A portion of them are absorbed from the gut and could increase the risk of chronic disease developing over a long period of time. The presence of excessive amounts of antioxidants markedly reduced the levels of toxins formed during digestion and thereby reduced the risk of chronic disease development. Thus it is clear that unabsorbed antioxidants perform a very useful function in reducing the levels of mutagens and carcinogens formed during the digestion of food.

SOLUBILITY OF ANTIOXIDANTS
AND POLYPHENOLIC COMPOUNDS

The lipid-soluble antioxidants include vitamin A, vitamin E, carotenoids, coenzyme Q10, and L-carnitine. Water-soluble antioxidants include vitamin C, glutathione, and alpha-lipoic acid. Polyphenolic compounds are generally fat-soluble. Fat-soluble vitamins and polyphenolic compounds should be taken with meals so that they are more readily absorbed.

AVAILABILITY OF ANTIOXIDANTS

Vitamin A
Vitamin A is commercially sold as retinyl palmitate, retinyl acetate, and retinoic acid and its analogs. Retinyl acetate or retinyl palmitate is converted to retinol in the intestine before absorption. Retinol is converted to retinoic acid in the cells. Retinoic acid performs all of the functions of vitamin A except for maintaining good vision. Retinol is stored in the liver as retinyl palmitate. Vitamin A exists as a protein-bound molecule. The level of retinol can be determined in the plasma.

Vitamin C
Vitamin C is commercially sold as ascorbic acid, sodium ascorbate, magnesium ascorbate, calcium ascorbate, and timed-release capsules containing ascorbic acid and vitamin C-ester. It is present in all cells. Ascorbic acid is converted to dehydroascorbic acid, which can be reduced to form vitamin C. It's interesting to note that dehydroascorbic acid can cross the blood-brain barrier, but vitamin C cannot. All

mammals make vitamin C except guinea pigs. An adult goat makes about thirteen grams of vitamin C every day. The plasma level of vitamin C may not reflect the tissue level of vitamin C, but in humans it's difficult to obtain tissues in order to determine vitamin C levels. Vitamin C can recycle oxidized vitamin E to the reduced form, which acts as an antioxidant.

Carotenoids

Beta-carotene is one of more than six hundred carotenoids found in fruits, vegetables, and plants. It is commercially available in natural or synthetic forms. The natural form of beta-carotene is more effective than the synthetic form. Preparations of natural carotenoids contain primarily beta-carotene; however, the other type of carotenoid is also present. A portion of ingested beta-carotene is converted to retinol (vitamin A) in the intestinal tract before absorption, and the remainder is distributed in the blood and tissues of the body. One molecule of beta-carotene forms two molecules of vitamin A. In humans the conversion of beta-carotene to vitamin A doesn't occur if the body has sufficient amounts of vitamin A. Beta-carotene is primarily stored in the eyes and fatty tissues. Other carotenoids such as lycopene accumulate in the prostate more than in any other organ, whereas lutein accumulates in the eyes more than in any other organ.

Coenzyme Q10

About 95 percent of energy is generated from the use of coenzyme Q10 by the mitochondria. Therefore, organs such as the heart and liver that require high energy have the highest concentrations of coenzyme Q10. Other organelles inside the cells that contain coenzyme Q10 include endoplasmic reticulum, peroxisomes, lysosomes, and Golgi apparatus.

Vitamin E

Among vitamin E isomers alpha-tocopherol is biologically more active than others. In recent years the research on tocotrienols has revealed some important biological functions. Vitamin E is commercially sold as d- or dl-tocopherol, alpha-tocopheryl acetate (alpha-TA), or alpha-tocopheryl succinate (alpha-TS). The esterified forms of vitamin E (alpha-TA and alpha-TS) are more stable than alpha-tocopherol. Alpha-TA has been widely used in basic research and clinical studies.

It's been presumed that alpha-TA or alpha-TS is converted to alpha-tocopherol in the intestinal tract before absorption. This assumption may be true for alpha-TS. If the body's stores of alpha-tocopherol are saturated, alpha-TS can be absorbed as alpha-TS. Alpha-TS enters the cells more easily than alpha-tocopherol because of its greater solubility. As well, alpha-TS has some unique functions that cannot be produced by alpha-T.

Alpha-TS is now considered the most effective form of vitamin E, but it cannot act as an antioxidant until converted to alpha-T. Alpha-T is located primarily in the membranous structures of the cells. The level of vitamin E can be determined in the plasma.

Glutathione and Alpha-Lipoic Acid

Glutathione is the most important antioxidant within the cells, and it is present in all cells. Although it's sold commercially for oral consumption, it's totally destroyed in the intestine. Therefore, oral administration of glutathione doesn't increase the cellular level of glutathione; however, N-acetylcysteine (NAC) does. In the body N-acetyl is removed from NAC by the enzyme esterase, and then cysteine is used to synthesize glutathione.

Alpha-lipoic acid also increases the cellular levels of glutathione by a mechanism that differs from the mechanism of NAC.

L-carnitine

L-carnitine is made in the body, but we can also obtain it from the diet. The highest concentration of L-carnitine is found in red meat (95 milligrams per 3.0 ounces of meat). In contrast, the chicken breast has only

3.9 milligrams per 3.5 ounces. L-carnitine is present in all of the cells of our body.

Melatonin

Melatonin is a naturally occurring hormone produced primarily by the pineal gland in the brain. It is also produced by the retina, the lens, and the gastrointestinal tract. Melatonin is synthesized from the amino acid tryptophan. It is also present in various plants such as rice. It is readily absorbed from the intestinal tract; however, 50 percent of it is removed from the plasma in thirty-five to fifty minutes. It has several biological functions including antioxidant and anti-inflammatory activities. Melatonin is necessary for the proper regulation of sleep cycles.

Nicotinamide (Vitamin B$_3$) and Nicotinamide Adenine Dinucleotide Dehydrogenase (NADH)

Treatment with nicotinamide, a precursor of nicotinamide adenine dinucleotide (NAD$^+$), reduced oxidative-stress-induced mitochondrial dysfunction and increased the survival of neurons in culture. Nicotinamide also attenuated glutamate-induced toxicity. Histone deacetylase inhibitors increase histone acetylation and enhance memory and neuronal plasticity. Nicotinamide (vitamin B$_3$), an inhibitor of histone deacetylase activity, restored memory deficits in Alzheimer's transgenic mice. Thus, the addition of nicotinamide at doses higher than recommended by RDA to a preparation of micronutrients may be necessary in order to reduce the risk of developing memory loss and to increase the survival of neurons in neurodegenerative diseases.

Nicotinamide adenine dinucleotide (NAD+) and NADH (the reduced form of NAD) are present in all of the cells of our body. NAD+ is an oxidizing agent; therefore, it can act as a pro-oxidant, whereas NADH can act as an antioxidant. NAD+ accepts electron from other molecules and is reduced to form NADH. NADH can recycle oxidized vitamin E to the reduced form, which can act as an antioxidant. NADH is essential for mitochondria to generate energy.

Polyphenolic Compounds

Flavonoids (polyphenolic compounds) are poorly absorbed by the intestinal tract in humans. All of them possess varying degrees of antioxidants and anti-inflammatory activities.

HOW TO STORE
ANTIOXIDANTS

Vitamin A

Crystal forms of retinol, retinoic acid, retinyl acetate, and retinal palmitate can be stored at 4°C for several months. A solution of retinoic acid is stable at 4°C, stored away from light, for several weeks.

Vitamin C

Vitamin C should not be stored in solution form because it is easily destroyed within a few days. The crystal or tablet forms of vitamin C can be kept at room temperature, away from light, for a few years.

Carotenoids

Most commercially sold carotenoids in solid form can be stored at room temperature, away from light, for a few years. Beta-carotene in solution, however, degrades within a few days, even when stored in a colder environment away from light.

Coenzyme Q10 and NADH

These antioxidants in solid forms are stable when stored at room temperature, away from light, for a few years. The solutions of these antioxidants are stable when stored at 4°C, away from light, for several months.

Vitamin E

Alpha-tocopherol is relatively unstable at room temperature in comparison to alpha-tocopheryl acetate and alpha-tocopheryl succinate. Alpha tocopherol can be stored at 4°C for several weeks, but alpha-tocopheryl acetate and alpha-tocopheryl succinate can be stored at room temperature for a few years. A solution of alpha-tocopheryl succinate is stable for several months at 4°C if kept away from the light.

Glutathione, N-acetylcysteine, and Alpha-Lipoic Acid

Solid forms of glutathione, N-acetylcysteine, and alpha-lipoic acid are stable at room temperature away from light, for a few years. The solutions of these antioxidants are stable when stored at 4°C, away from light, for several months.

Melatonin

The powdered form of melatonin is stable at 4°C for a year or more.

Polyphenolic Compounds

Polyphenolic compounds are very stable at room temperature, away from light, for a few years.

CAN ANTIOXIDANTS BE DESTROYED DURING COOKING?

Vitamin A

Routine cooking does not destroy vitamin A, but slow heating for a long period of time may reduce its potency. Canning and prolonged cold storage may also diminish its activity. The vitamin A content of fortified milk powder declines substantially after two years.

Carotenoids

Most carotenes, especially lutein and lycopene, are not destroyed during cooking. In fact, their bioavailability improves when they're derived from a cooked or extracted preparation, for example, lycopene from tomato sauce.

Coenzyme Q10 and NADH

Coenzyme Q10 and NADH can be partially degraded during cooking.

Vitamin E

Food processing, frying, and freezing destroy vitamin E. The vitamin E content of fortified milk powder is unaffected over a two-year period.

Glutathione, N-acetylcysteine, and Alpha-Lipoic Acid

Glutathione, N-acetylcysteine, and alpha-lipoic acid can be partially destroyed during cooking.

Polyphenolic Compounds

Polylphenolic compounds are not destroyed during cooking.

CONCLUDING REMARKS

Early in the mists of time, when life on the planet consisted primarily of small anaerobic organisms, oxygen as we know it today did not yet exist. However, these organisms eventually acquired the ability to break water down into its constituent parts of hydrogen and oxygen. This oxygen was a toxic substance, and thus, the few forms of life that existed had to adapt to it in order to survive. They did this by developing antioxidant defensive systems that would protect them from oxidative damage. As these organisms evolved into humans, the defensive antioxidant shields evolved with them.

When the body processes oxygen, free radicals are created. Infection and metabolism are two additional processes that generate free radicals in the body. As well, certain trace minerals (iron, copper, and manganese, in combination with molecules like vitamin C and uric acid) can also form free radicals. These free radicals may threaten to overwhelm the body's antioxidant system, thus underscoring the need to ensure the presence of large amounts of antioxidants in the body at all times.

There are many different types of antioxidants, both those that are made in the body and those that are derived from outside sources via either diet or dietary supplement. In terms of dietary antioxidants and guidance regarding the same, it's useful to refer to the Daily Recommended Intake, which is an index established for each micronutrient. The DRI is found in the appendix of this book. (The DRI replaces the former index known as the Recommended Dietary Allowance.) However, and it must be noted, that although these recommended doses allow for normal growth and development, they're not optimal for reducing increased oxidative stress and inflammation.

In the next chapter we will examine the role of antioxidants in reducing chronic inflammation and increased oxidative stress by looking at how antioxidants are currently perceived by the medical community and how they are being utilized in studies designed to further explore the causative factors of Alzheimer's disease.

5
The Role of Antioxidants in Reducing Oxidative Damage

Despite the fact antioxidants are so essential for our growth and survival, they remain misunderstood by most public health and health care professionals. As a result their true potential is infrequently realized. The reasons for this include inaccurate claims by many in the nutrition industry, inconsistent human data (stemming from epidemiologic studies), and the results of poorly designed clinical studies in which one or a few dietary antioxidants were administered to populations at high risk for the development of chronic disease.

This chapter outlines current controversies about the value of micronutrients for disease prevention and the misuse of antioxidants in clinical studies for the prevention of chronic diseases. More information about the role of nuclear transcription factor-2 (Nrf2) in reducing oxidative stress, inflammation, and glutamate release and toxicity is also included.

MISCONCEPTIONS ABOUT ANTIOXIDANTS

Basic scientific evidence exists that validates both the significance of multiple antioxidants when used in combination with standard therapy for disease prevention and the value of multiple antioxidants in the management of chronic disease. And yet the medical establishment remains skeptical on both points. It should be noted that this is not the first time the medical community has failed to acknowledge the value of multiple antioxidants in these contexts. As we have established earlier the cure for night blindness and scurvy was delayed for centuries because of reluctance on the part of the medical community to embrace cures that were deemed to be not in keeping with the traditional models.

Be this as it may, before we can completely understand the flaws inherent in current methodologies pertaining to antioxidant supplementation, we need to know a bit more about free radicals. The human body generates different types of inorganic and organic free radicals derived from oxygen and nitrogen in response to the utilization of oxygen. Exposure to various environmental stressors such as ozone, dust particles, smoke, toxic fumes, toxic chemicals, and ionizing radiation (X-rays or gamma rays), also produces excessive amounts of free radicals in the body. Free-radical-induced damage is called oxidative damage, which also occurs during the normal aging process and during the initiation and progression of certain neurodegenerative diseases.

An elevation of dietary and endogenous antioxidant chemicals as well as antioxidant enzymes simultaneously is needed to reduce oxidative stress and inflammation optimally. I propose that supplementation with a preparation of micronutrients containing dietary and endogenous antioxidants, B vitamins, vitamin D, selenium, and certain phenolic compounds (curcumin and resveratrol) may be essential for reducing *the risk of developing* as well as *of slowing* the progression of Alzheimer's disease. This preparation would increase the levels of antioxidant enzymes and the levels of dietary and endogenous antioxidant chemicals at the same time. Unfortunately, as we know, nearly all previous clinical studies have utilized just one or two dietary antioxidants in populations that are at a high risk of developing certain chronic diseases, thus yielding inconsistent results. Let's now look at some other factors that are important to consider when undertaking the design of a clinical study.

OPTIMAL TYPES AND DOSES OF ANTIOXIDANTS

When designing a human clinical study, the *type* of antioxidant employed is key. For example, it's been reported that natural beta-carotene prevented the X-ray-induced transformation of normal mouse fibroblasts in culture, whereas synthetic beta-carotene did not. An animal study showed that various organs accumulated the natural form of vitamin E (d-alpha-tocopherol) more than the synthetic form (dl-alpha-tocopherol). Furthermore, it has been reported that vitamin E in the form of d-alpha-tocopheryl succinate is more effective than other forms of vitamin E. Human studies with antioxidants have not taken these important issues into consideration; therefore, results pertaining to the efficacy of antioxidants have been contradictory.

The *doses* of antioxidants utilized are also very important in preventing disease and producing optimal health benefits. Low doses (those approximating DRI/RDA values) may be useful in reducing some oxidative damage and preventing deficiency. However, they may not be sufficient in reducing inflammation or optimizing immune function. The differences in changes in the expression of gene profiles between low and high doses of an antioxidant are very marked. In commercially sold multivitamin preparations, the dose amounts of antioxidants and other micronutrients vary markedly.

The *dose-schedule* of antioxidant micronutrients is also very critical in achieving the desired health benefits. Most people take micronutrient supplements once a day, which may not produce an optimal result. This is due to the fact that there is a high degree of fluctuation in the levels of antioxidants in the body because of a variation in the plasma half-lives of different micronutrients. In addition, as noted above, the expression of cell gene profiles differs markedly, depending on the level of antioxidants in the body. A once-a-day dose-schedule may compel the cells to constantly adjust their genetic activity due to variations in antioxidant levels in the body. Such a large fluctuation in genetic activity may not be desirable for optimal cell functioning. It's interesting to note that all previous human studies with antioxidants have utilized this once-a-day dose-schedule in spite of scientific evidence indicating that this is far from ideal.

In all human studies with antioxidants, the selection of the target population and the statistical analyses have been appropriate, but the selection of antioxidants, their doses and dose-schedule, have been designed without any real scientific rationale. This can be demonstrated by an examination of some widely publicized results of antioxidant studies as follows.

FLAWED ANTIOXIDANT STUDIES IN HUMANS

In a clinical study the synthetic form of beta-carotene was administered orally once a day, to males who were heavy tobacco smokers, in order to reduce the incidence of lung cancer. The results showed that the incidence of lung cancer in smokers who were treated with beta-carotene increased by about 17 percent (Albanes et al. 1995). Federal agencies and some nutrition scientists then promoted the idea that supplementation with beta-carotene may be harmful to one's health and recommended that consumers not take beta-carotene in any form or in any multivitamin preparation. These erroneous conclusions and recommendations were without any scientific merit for the following reasons.

It had been known before the start of this particular study that individual antioxidants such as beta-carotene can be oxidized in a high oxidative environment to become a pro-oxidant. Heavy tobacco smokers have a high internal oxidative environment. Therefore, when beta-carotene is administered to smokers, it is oxidized and acts as a pro-oxidant rather than as an antioxidant. Thus the expected outcome *would be* an increase in the incidence of cancer in tobacco smokers.

In contrast to the adverse effects of beta-carotene in heavy tobacco smokers, the same dose and type of beta-carotene did not increase the incidence of cancer among doctors and nurses who were nonsmokers during a five-year follow-up (Hennekens et al. 1996). Again, this result was also expected because populations of nonsmokers do not have a high internal oxidative environment.

Studies have also been done utilizing only vitamin E. Studies utilizing its synthetic and natural forms have produced inconsistent results in patients at high risk for the development of cardiovascular disease who also have an elevated internal oxidative environment. Some studies showed beneficial effects, whereas others showed no effect—or even adverse effects in some cases (Tornwall et al. 2004a; Tornwall et al. 2004b; Leppala et al. 2000; Yusuf et al. 2000).

The harmful effects of vitamin E alone on cardiovascular disease can be attributed to the same biological events as those observed with beta-carotene. At this time cardiologists do not recommend vitamin E to their patients. There are no human data (intervention studies) to show that the same dose of vitamin E or beta-carotene, when present in an appropriately prepared multivitamin formula that includes dietary and endogenous antioxidants, produces adverse health effects among normal or high-risk populations.

Human studies featuring a single antioxidant have also produced inconsistent results in neurological diseases such as Parkinson's disease and Alzheimer's. In both studies high doses of the synthetic form of vitamin E (800 IU per day in the case of Parkinson's and 2,000 IU per day in the case of Alzheimer's) were used. No beneficial effects of vitamin E were observed in the study involving Parkinson's disease (Shoulson et al. 1998), but some beneficial effects were observed in the study pertaining to Alzheimer's disease (Sano et al. 1997). These studies were undertaken without a careful consideration of the biochemical factors involved in the disease processes or the antioxidant status of the patients involved.

It's been reported that a deficiency of the antioxidant glutathione is found in patients with Alzheimer's and Parkinson's disease. In addition, dysfunction of the mitochondria is consistently observed in the autopsied brains of patients with Parkinson's and Alzheimer's. Evidence of high oxidative damage and chronic inflammation have also been found in the brains of these patients. Therefore, the idea of supplementation with antioxidants to prevent or reduce the rate of progression of these diseases is an idea with merit. Supplementation with a multiple micronutrient preparation that contains appropriate doses of dietary, endogenous antioxidants and certain polyphenolic compounds that would increase the levels of antioxidant enzymes by activating a nuclear transcriptional factor Nrf2 and antioxidant chemicals at the same time would be useful in optimally reducing the oxidaitive stress and chronic inflammation.

It's very unfortunate that the harmful results obtained with the use of primarily one antioxidant in high-risk populations are often extrapolated to all multiple antioxidant preparations and all populations. This erroneous extrapolation of data regarding the harmful effects of beta-carotene or vitamin E alone, for instance, is further propagated by the publication of meta-analysis of published data on the same vitamins with the same conclusion. A meta-analysis publication is often misinterpreted to be an original study. In my opinion a meta-analysis should critically examine an experiment's design instead of just summarizing various study results.

Due to the fact that these studies are so poorly and inconsistently designed, their extrapolations have created a wide disconnect between the public and most health care professionals—especially physicians—regarding the health benefits of micronutrients. In an attempt to rectify this misunderstanding, in the subsequent chapters of this book, I discuss the scientific basis for utilizing multiple micronutrients, including dietary and endogenous antioxidants, to reduce the risk of development and progression of Alzheimer's disease. In addition, the role of these micronutrients in improving the efficacy of standard therapy in Alzheimer's disease is also discussed.

THE REDUCTION OF OXIDATIVE STRESS, CHRONIC INFLAMMATION, AND GLUTAMATE RELEASE IN THE BRAIN

As we know significant studies have suggested that increased oxidative stress and chronic inflammation are involved in the development and progression of Alzheimer's disease. Glutamate release in the extracellular space of the brain occurs at the late stage of this disease. Therefore, reducing the levels of these biologically harmful processes may prevent the development and progression of Alzheimer's disease and, in combination with standard therapy, may improve its management.

How to Reduce Oxidative Stress

Increased oxidative stress in the brain can be most effectively reduced by increasing the levels of antioxidant enzymes, as well as by elevating the levels of dietary and endogenous antioxidant chemicals at the same time. They work by different mechanisms. For example, antioxidant enzymes reduce free radicals by catalysis (converting them into harmless molecules by a chemical reaction), whereas dietary and endogenous antioxidant chemicals reduce free radicals by scavenging them directly.

As mentioned previously, in response to reactive oxygen species (ROS), a nuclear transcriptional factor, Nrf2 (nuclear factor-erythroid 2-related factor 2), translocates from the cytoplasm to the nucleus where it binds with antioxidant response elements (ARE), which increases the levels of antioxidant enzymes in order to reduce oxidative damage (Itoh et al. 1997; Hayes et al. 2000; Chan, Han, and Kan 2001). In response to increased oxidative stress, existing levels of dietary and endogenous antioxidant chemicals levels cannot be elevated without supplementation.

Factors Regulating Response of Nrf2 and Its Action

Several studies exist to support the conclusion that antioxidant enzymes are elevated by Nrf2 activation through ROS-dependent (Niture et al. 2010) and independent mechanisms (Xi et al. 2012; Li et al. 2012; Bergstrom et al. 2011; Wruck et al. 2008; Hine and Mitchell 2012).

As part of this process the levels of antioxidant enzymes are also dependent upon the binding ability of Nrf2 with ARE in the nucleus (Suh et al. 2004).

Differential Response of Nrf2 to ROS
Generated during Acute and Chronic Oxidative Stress

In terms of ROS production it appears that Nrf2 responds differently to *acute* oxidative stress than it does to *chronic* oxidative stress. For example, excessive amounts of ROS are generated during the acute oxidative stress observed in an individual undergoing strenuous exercise. In response to the increased ROS, as we know, Nrf2 translocates from the cytoplasm to the nucleus where it binds with ARE to upregulate antioxidant genes. Excessive amounts of ROS are also present during chronic oxidative stress commonly found in older individuals and in individuals with neurological diseases such as Parkinson's disease, Alzheimer's disease, and post-traumatic stress disorder, suggesting that the Nrf2/ARE regulatory system has become unresponsive to ROS in these diseases. Age-related decline in antioxidant enzymes in the liver of older rats compared to that in younger rats was due to reduction in the binding ability of Nrf2 with ARE. However, treatment with alpha-lipoic acid restored this defect, increased the levels of antioxidant enzymes, and restored the loss of glutathione from the liver of old rats (Suh et al. 2004). The exact reasons for the Nrf2/ARE regulatory system to become unresponsive to ROS during chronic oxidative stress are unknown. However, defects in the binding ability of Nrf2 with ARE may be part of the answer.

The levels of Nrf2 in the nucleus decreased in the hippocampal neurons of patients with Alzheimer's despite increased oxidative stress (Ramsey et al. 2007). In addition, an activation of Nrf2 in Alzheimer's disease also becomes unresponsive to ROS stimulation. It is also possible that the Nrf2 binding ability with ARE is impaired. It is not known whether the defect in the Nrf2 pathway occurs in the cytoplasm where Nrf2 forms a complex with INrf2 (an inhibitor of Nrf2) or at the level of the nucleus where it binds with ARE to enhance the expression of antioxidant genes—or at both levels.

Treatment with tert-butylhydroquinone, a known inducer of Nrf2, protected neurons against beta-amyloid-induced damage to the nerve cells in transgenic Alzheimer's mice. Insertion of the Nrf2 gene into the nerve cells protected them from the damaging effects of beta-amyloids (Kanninen et al. 2008).

The following groups of agents demonstrate that some antioxidant chemicals and polyphenolic compounds may have a dual function given that they decrease oxidative stress by increasing antioxidant enzymes through activating the Nrf2/ARE pathway as well as directly by scavenging free radicals, whereas others scavenge free radicals directly. These agents are listed here.

1. **Free radical scavenging antioxidants:** All dietary and endogenous antioxidant chemicals reduce varying levels of oxidative stress by directly scavenging free radicals. Some examples are dietary antioxidants—such as vitamin A, beta-carotene, vitamin C, vitamin E, and polyphenolic compounds—and endogenous antioxidants, such as glutathione, alpha-lipoic acid, and coenzyme Q10.

2. **Antioxidants activating Nrf2 by a ROS-independent mechanism:** Some examples are the organosulfur compound sulforaphane, found in cruciferous vegetables; kavalactones, found in kava shrubs; and puerarin, a major flavonoid from the root of *Pueraria lobata* (Bergstrom et al. 2011; Wruck et al. 2008; Zou et al. 2013). Genistein and vitamin E (Xi et al. 2012) and coenzyme Q10 (Choi et al. 2009) also activate Nrf2 by a ROS-independent mechanism.

3. **Antioxidants scavenging free radicals as well as activation by a ROS-independent mechanism:** Some examples are vitamin E (Xi et al. 2012), alpha-lipoic acid (Suh et al. 2004), curcumin (Trujillo et al. 2013), resveratrol (Steele et al. 2013, Kode et al. 2008), omega-3 fatty acids (Gao et al. 2007; Saw et al. 2013), and NAC (Ji et al. 2010).

4. **Antioxidant activating Nrf2 by a ROS-dependent mechanism:** L-carnitine activates Nrf2 by a ROS-dependent mechanism (Zambrano et al. 2013). This could have been due to the generation of transient ROS by L-carnitine.

A combination of selected agents from the above groups may reduce oxidative stress optimally, and thereby may reduce the risk of developing Alzheimer's disease, and in combination with standard therapy, may improve the management of this disease.

How to Reduce Chronic Inflammation and Glutamate Release

Some individual antioxidants from the groups above have been shown to reduce chronic inflammation (Abate et al. 2000; Devaraj et al. 2007; Fu et al. 2008; Lee et al. 2007; Peairs and Rankin 2008; Rahman et al. 2008; Suzuki, Aggarwal, and Packer 1992; Zhu et al. 2008). They have also been shown to prevent the release (Barger et al. 2007) and toxicity of glutamate (Schubert, Kimura, and Maher 1992; Sandhu et al. 2003). A combination of selected agents from the groups above may reduce chronic inflammation and the release of glutamate and its toxicity optimally. In so doing it may thereby reduce the risk of developing Alzheimer's disease and, in combination with standard therapy, may improve the management of this disease.

CONCLUDING REMARKS

Micronutrients include antioxidants, B vitamins, vitamin D, and selenium. Macronutrients include protein, carbohydrate, and fat. However, only the properties and functions of antioxidants and polyphenolic compounds have been described in this chapter. Certain antioxidants are consumed through the diet, and others are made in the body. Polyphenolic compounds are consumed exclusively through the diet. Some dietary and endogenous antioxidant chemicals and polyphenolic compounds reduce oxidative stress by directly scavenging free radicals, whereas others reduce it by elevating antioxidant enzymes through the activation of Nrf2/ARE pathway.

Several of these agents have a dual function because they can activate the ROS-independent Nrf2/ARE pathway for increasing antioxidant enzymes and scavenge free radicals directly. Therefore, selected agents from these groups of antioxidants at appropriate doses may be necessary for the prevention and improved management of Alzheimer's disease. Unfortunately, clinical studies with antioxidants in a population at high risk of developing chronic diseases have utilized a single antioxidant or only a few. The results of these studies have been inconsistent.

A separate preparation of micronutrients, including dietary and endogenous antioxidants and certain polyphenolic compounds (curcumin and resveratrol), employed to reduce the risk of Alzheimer's disease, will be proposed in subsequent chapters. These agents are capable of reducing oxidative stress, chronic inflammation, and the release and toxicity of glutamate by increasing antioxidant enzyme levels through the activation of the Nrf2/ARE pathway, as well as by scavenging free radicals directly.

6 Laboratory and Clinical Studies of Antioxidants and Alzheimer's Symptoms

Despite extensive research and the publication of thousands of research studies on the causes of Alzheimer's disease, it has not been possible to reduce its incidence or rate of progression. As established in the previous chapter, the medical community has a flawed understanding of the true value of antioxidants in this regard, and as a result studies utilizing antioxidants have not taken advantage of their full preventive and therapeutic potentials.

Several laboratory studies have demonstrated that treatment with individual dietary antioxidants, endogenous antioxidants, B vitamins, omega-3 fatty acids, and certain polyphenolic compounds protected nerve cells and improved some symptoms in animal Alzheimer's models and also in nerve cell culture. A few clinical studies with an individual antioxidant have produced inconsistent results in patients with mild to moderate Alzheimer's. No studies have been performed with a preparation of micronutrients containing multiple antioxidants and certain polyphenolic compounds (curcumin and resveratrol), which can activate the Nrf2/ARE pathway and increase the levels of dietary and endogenous antioxidant chemicals in the body at the same time.

This chapter describes laboratory studies and clinical studies done on oxidative stress and some symptoms of Alzheimer's utilizing individual agents (antioxidants, B vitamins, omega-3 fatty acids, and polyphenolic compounds). In addition, the reasons for inconsistent results obtained from the use of a single micronutrient in human Alzheimer's studies, but not in animal models of the disease, are also explored.

THE LABORATORY STUDIES

Laboratory Studies with Alpha-Lipoic Acid

One particular laboratory study (Alzheimer's model) involved the use of nerve cell culture and transgenic Alzheimer's animal models. The fibroblasts from Alzheimer's disease patients exhibited the highest levels of markers of oxidative damage in comparison to the fibroblasts from age-matched and healthy individuals. However, treatment with alpha-lipoic acid and N-acetylcysteine individually reduced the levels of markers of oxidative damage; the combination of the two was more effective than the individual agents (Moreira et al. 2007).

Alpha-lipoic acid treatment also reduced beta-amyloid-induced damage to the nerve cells in culture (Zhang et al. 2001). The natural form of alpha-lipoic acid (R-LA) was more effective than the synthetic form (Rac-LA) (Carlson et al. 2007).

In a mouse model of Alzheimer's disease, administration of R-LA through the diet reduced oxidative damage but did not improve cognitive performance or the levels of beta-amyloids (Siedlak et al. 2009). On the other hand chronic administration of alpha-lipoic acid through diet improved the memory of transgenic Alzheimer's mice model (Quinn et al. 2007).

Pretreatment of transgenic Alzheimer's mice (SAMP8) with alpha-lipoic acid enhanced memory function and learning ability by increasing glutathione levels and glutathione peroxidase activity and decreasing malondialdehyde (MDA) levels (Farr et al. 2012). Efficacy of alpha-lipoic acid in improving cognitive function differs even in animal

Alzheimer's models, depending on the type of Alzheimer's model used.

Dietary supplementation with a combination of alpha-lipoic acid, acetyl-L-carnitine, glycerophosphocoline, docosahexaenoic acid, and phosphatidylserine reduced oxidative damage in the mouse brain and improved cognitive performance (Suchy, Chan, and Shea 2009).

Treatment with a new conjugate molecule of ibuprofen-lipoic acid enhanced the levels of neuroglobin (a neuroprotective protein in the brain) and decreased the loss of nerve cells in transgenic Alzheimer's model rats (Zara et al. 2013).

Alpha-lipoic acid protects nerve cells against oxidative damage in the following ways:

1. It increases acetylcholine levels by increasing choline acetyltransferase activity. Since acetylcholine is involved in memory, elevated levels of acetylcholine may improve memory.
2. It removes certain metals, such as copper, iron, zinc, and aluminum. Removal of excessive amounts of these metals from the brain is necessary because each of them combines with beta-amyloids and forms aggregates. The aggregated form of beta-amyloids is toxic to the nerve cells.
3. It directly scavenges free radicals.
4. It increases glutathione levels (Holmquist et al. 2007).
5. It reduces the expression of pro-inflammatory cytokines such as TNF-alpha and inducible nitric oxide synthase (iNOS) (Maczurek et al. 2008).

Laboratory Studies with Caffeine

Long-term caffeine consumption decreased the production of beta-amyloids and improved cognitive function in Alzheimer's transgenic mice. Therefore, it was suggested that moderate daily consumption of caffeine may reduce the risk of Alzheimer's disease (Arendash et al. 2006). No studies to evaluate the effectiveness of caffeine alone in reducing the risk of developing Alzheimer's in humans have been performed.

Laboratory Studies with Coenzyme Q10

Coenzyme Q10 reduced overproduction of beta-amyloids and intra-cellular deposits of beta-amyloids in the cortex region of the brain in Alzheimer's transgenic mice (Yang et al. 2008). In addition, coenzyme Q10 treatment decreased malondialdehyde (MDA) levels and enhanced the activity of SOD in these mice.

It has been reported that supplementation with both coenzyme Q10 and alpha-tocopheryl acetate improved age-related learning deficits in mice (McDonald, Sohal, and Forster 2005). Coenzyme Q10 also prevented the formation of beta-amyloid fibrils and destabilized preformed beta-amyloid aggregates (Ono et al. 2005). It also decreased beta-amyloid-induced mitochondrial dysfunction in vitro (Moreira et al. 2005).

No well-designed human studies to evaluate the effectiveness of coenzyme Q10 in reducing the development or progression of Alzheimer's disease have been performed.

Laboratory Studies with Curcumin

Curcumin is a natural yellow pigment of turmeric that is widely used as a spice throughout the Indian subcontinent. It exhibits antioxidant and anti-inflammatory activities. Curcumin treatment inhibits the aggregation of beta-amyloids in vitro.

Curcumin prevented an aluminum-induced aggregation of beta-amyloids and its toxicity on rat neuronal cells in culture (Jiang et al. 2012). Preparation of curcumin-liposome was also very effective in reducing the aggregation of beta-amyloids and the oligomer formation of beta-amyloids (Taylor et al. 2011). In an animal model of Alzheimer's disease, curcumin reduced aggregation of beta-amyloids and the formation of oligomers of beta-amyloids and phosphorylation of tau protein (Hamaguchi et al. 2010).

Laboratory Studies with Edaravone

Edaravone (3-methyl-1-phenyl-2-pyrazolin-5-one) is a synthetic drug widely used for the treatment of cerebral infarction in Japan and other countries. Edaravone exhibits powerful antioxidant activity. Pretreatment of rat neuroblastoma cells (PC-12 cell line) with Edaravone increased glutathione levels and SOD activity and decreased MDA levels and beta-amyloid aggregation (Zhang et al. 2013).

The toxicity of this drug after long-term consumption in humans is unknown. To be used in patients with Alzheimer's disease would require the approval of the Food and Drug Administration.

Laboratory Studies with Genistein

Genistein is an active ingredient of soybean isoflavone. Treatment with genistein prevented Aß-25-35-induced mitochondrial DNA damage in glioma cells (C-6) (Ma et al. 2013) and oxidative damage in rat neuroblastoma cells (Xi et al. 2011).

No studies to evaluate the effectiveness of genistein in reducing the risk of Alzheimer's in humans have been performed.

Laboratory Studies with Ginkgo Biloba

Long-term consumption of ginkgo biloba extract through diet lowered APP levels by 50 percent in the cortex region of the brain of transgenic Alzheimer's mice compared to that of normal mice (Augustin et al. 2009).

Laboratory Studies with Green Tea Epigallocatechin-3-gallate (EGCG)

Treatment of transgenic Alzheimer's mice with green tea epigallocatechin-3-gallate (EGCG) improved cognitive function and reduced the levels of beta-amyloids and hyperphosphorylated tau protein (Rezai-Zadeh et al. 2008). Pretreatment of transgenic (Tg) Alzheimer's mice with green tea catechin (GTC) reduced the production of beta-amyloids and degenerative changes in the nerve cells of the brain (Lim et al. 2013).

No studies to evaluate the effectiveness of EGCG alone in reducing the risk of developing Alzheimer's disease in humans have been performed.

Laboratory Studies with Melatonin

Melatonin treatment increased the levels of thiobarbituric acid–reactive substances (TBARS), SOD activity, and glutathione levels in Alzheimer's transgenic mice (Feng et al. 2006).

Long-term melatonin treatment improved cognitive function in Alzheimer's transgenic mice. The mechanisms of this protection by melatonin involve preventing the aggregation of beta-amyloids and reducing the levels of pro-inflammatory cytokines and oxidative stress (Olcese et al. 2009).

These studies suggest that treatment with melatonin alone may be useful in improving some symptoms of Alzheimer's disease by reducing oxidative stress and chronic inflammation in the animal Alzheimer's model.

Laboratory Studies with Resveratrol

Resveratrol, a major polyphenol in red wine, exhibits neuroprotective effects in vitro and in animal models (Vingtdeux et al. 2008; Wang et al. 2006).

Resveratrol protects neuronal cells in culture against beta-amyloid-induced toxicity. This effect is mediated through enhancing the intracellular levels of glutathione, an important antioxidant within the cells (Savaskan et al. 2003). It also lowered the intracellular levels of beta-amyloids in different neuronal cell lines (Marambaud, Zhao, and Davies 2005).

This effect of resveratrol was due to increased degradation of beta-amyloids by proteasome. Resveratrol treatment of mouse astrocytes reduced lipopolysaccharide (LPS)-induced inflammation by decreasing the production of nitric oxide and the pro-inflammatory cytokines TNF-alpha, IL-6, IL-1beta, and C-reactive protein (markers of chronic inflammation) (Wight et al. 2012).

Resveratrol treatment reduced degeneration and death of the nerve cells in an animal model of Alzheimer's disease (Anekonda 2006).

Laboratory Studies with Selenium

Relatively large amounts of Selenoprotein M (SelM) are present in the human brain. Treatment with sodium selenite increased the levels of this protein, which acts as an antioxidant (Chen et al. 2013).

SelM and Selenoprotein P (SelP-H) inhibited zinc-induced beta-amyloid aggregation and beta-amyloid-induced ROS production in vitro (Du et al. 2013). The aggregated form of beta-amyloids is toxic to the nerve cells.

Laboratory Studies with Vitamin A or Beta-Carotene Alone

Vitamin A, or beta-carotene, inhibited the formation of beta-amyloid aggregates in a dose-dependent manner. They also destabilized pre-formed beta-amyloid aggregates in vitro (Ono et al. 2004). These effects of vitamins A and beta-carotene may reduce the toxicity of beta-amyloids on the nerve cells in culture.

Treatment with retinoic acid, a metabolite of vitamin A, decreased the activation of microglia and astrocytes, reduced the degeneration of neurons, and improved spatial learning and memory in the Alzheimer's transgenic mice model compared to those mice not treated with retinoic acid (Ding et al. 2008).

Laboratory Studies with Vitamin B₃ (Nicotinamide)

Histone deacetylase inhibitors increase histone acetylation and thereby increase the activity of several genes. Treatment with an inhibitor of histone deacetylase enhances memory and the functional ability of neurons. Indeed, nicotinamide, an inhibitor histone deacetylase activity, restored memory deficits in Alzheimer's transgenic mice (Green et al. 2008). In addition, nicotinamide selectively reduced microtubule aggregation, which disrupts synaptic connections between neurons, leading to the death of nerve cells.

Nicotinamide also reduced glutamate-induced toxicity in nerve cells (Liu, Pitta, and Mattson 2008). In addition, treatment of transgenic

Alzheimer's model mice (3xTg) with nicotinamide improved cognitive function and reduced the levels of beta-amyloids and hyperphosphorylated tau as well as degeneration of the nerve cells (Liu et al. 2013).

These preclinical data suggest that oral supplementation with nicotinamide may be safe and useful in the management of Alzheimer's. No studies with nicotinamide alone or in combination with standard therapy in the management of patients with Alzheimer's disease have been performed.

Laboratory Studies
with Vitamin E and Pycnogenol

In Alzheimer's transgenic mice vitamin E supplementation reduced the levels and deposits of beta-amyloids in the brain; however, vitamin E supplementation was ineffective in decreasing the levels and deposits of amyloids in older mice (Sung et al. 2004).

Vitamin E treatment protected nerve cells of the hippocampus region of the brain against beta-amyloid-induced toxicity (Varadarajan et al. 1999). It also protected nerve cells in culture against beta-amyloid-induced toxicity (Behl et al. 1992).

Vitamin E and pycnogenol protected neuronal cells in culture against beta-amyloid-induced apoptosis by reducing caspase-3 activation and DNA damage (Peng, Buzzard, and Lau 2002).

Plasma phospholipid transfer protein (PLTP) transfers vitamin E from the plasma to the cells. Deficiency of the PLTP in mice would cause a reduction in the levels of vitamin E in the brain, which would increase oxidative stress. Indeed, removal of PLTP caused increased oxidative stress and increased beta-amyloid levels and decreased synaptic functioning in mice (Desrumaux et al. 2013). The administration of oligomers of beta-amyloid directly into the brain increased memory loss in PLTP-deleted mice.

Supplementation with vitamin E through diet prevented beta-amyloid oligomers-induced memory loss and reduced oxidative stress and degenerative changes in the brain (Desrumaux et al. 2013).

THE HUMAN STUDIES

Human Studies with Alpha-Lipoic Acid

In an open-label study involving forty-three patients with mild to moderate Alzheimer's disease receiving standard therapy, with a follow-up period of forty-eight months, it was observed that the addition of alpha-lipoic acid to the treatment protocol reduced the progression of the disease (Hager et al. 2007).

This effect was more pronounced in patients with mild Alzheimer's disease than in those with moderate Alzheimer's. No well-designed human studies to evaluate the effectiveness of alpha-lipoic acid alone in reducing the development or progression of Alzheimer's have been performed.

Human Studies with B Vitamins

In most studies the serum levels of vitamin B_{12} in Alzheimer's patients were lower than in normal healthy individuals (controls). Low levels of vitamin B_{12} may in part contribute to the degeneration of neurons in Alzheimer's patients (Cole and Prchal 1984). Indeed, vitamin B_{12} supplementation improved cognitive functions in Alzheimer's patients (Ikeda et al. 1992).

Supplementation with folic acid (vitamin B_9) improved the effectiveness of medication (cholinesterase inhibitor) in improving memory in patients with Alzheimer's disease (Malouf and Grimley Evans 2008).

In another multicenter human study supplementation with folic acid, vitamin B_6, and vitamin B_{12} did not reduce decline in cognitive function in individuals with mild to moderate Alzheimer's disease (Aisen et al. 2008).

Supplementation with vitamin B_{12} alone did not improve cognitive function or psychiatric symptoms in a vast majority of elderly patients with dementia having low serum vitamin B_{12} levels (van Dyck et al. 2009).

These studies suggest that treatment with one or more B vitamins did not produce consistent beneficial effects in patients with Alzheimer's disease.

Human Studies with Curcumin

Two clinical studies performed in the United States and China revealed no beneficial effect of curcumin on cognitive function in Alzheimer's patients compared to those Alzheimer's patients who received no curcumin (placebo) (Hamaguchi, Ono, and Yamada 2010).

These studies suggest that the use of curcumin alone in human Alzheimer's disease may be ineffective, even though it exhibits strong antioxidant and anti-inflammatory activities in laboratory experiments.

Human Studies with Ginkgo Biloba

A well-designed clinical trial among community volunteers age seventy-five or older with normal memory revealed that the administration of ginkgo biloba was not effective in reducing the incidence of Alzheimer's disease or overall dementia (DeKosky et al. 2008).

Human Studies with Vitamin E

An analysis of a few clinical studies revealed that vitamin E alone may not be useful in the prevention or treatment of Alzheimer's disease (Isaac, Quinn, and Tabet 2008; Farina et al. 2012).

However, a human clinical study with dl-alpha-tocopherol (the synthetic form of vitamin E; 2,000 IU per day) showed that the rate of decline in memory slowed down somewhat in patients with Alzheimer's (Sano et al. 1997).

Human Studies with Vitamin E and Vitamin C

In an epidemiologic study (survey-type study) among individuals with dementia age sixty-five and older, it was found that the use of vitamin C and vitamin E in combination was associated with a reduced incidence of Alzheimer's (Zandi et al. 2004).

In certain counties of North Carolina, a survey-type study was performed among older African Americans and white Americans from 1986 to 2000. The results revealed that these populations consumed fewer vitamin supplements than those living outside of these counties. However, the results also revealed that those individuals who consumed vitamin C and/or vitamin E did not show any effect on the incidence of Alzheimer's disease or dementia (from their vitamin consumption) (Fillenbaum et al. 2005).

In another survey-type of study performed by the Group Health Cooperative in Seattle, Washington, it was found that supplementation with vitamin E and vitamin C individually or in combination did not reduce the risk of Alzheimer's disease (Gray et al. 2008).

These studies suggest that treatment with one or two dietary antioxidants alone does not produce consistent results in patients with Alzheimer's.

In order to determine the antioxidant status in patients with Alzheimer's disease, serum and cerebrospinal fluid (CSF) levels of dietary antioxidants were determined. The results showed that serum levels of vitamin E and beta-carotene were lower in patients with Alzheimer's disease and other dementia compared to those of normal individuals (controls) (Zaman et al. 1992).

In another study serum levels of beta-carotene and vitamin A were lower in Alzheimer's patients compared to those of normal individuals; however, the levels of alpha-carotene did not change (Jimenez-Jimenez et al. 1999).

The average CSF and serum level of vitamin E was lower in patients with Alzheimer's disease than in normal individuals (Jimenez-Jimenez et al. 1997).

The plasma levels of dietary antioxidants (vitamin A, vitamin C, vitamin E, and carotenoids including beta-carotene, alpha-carotene, lutein, zeaxanthin, and lycopene) and the activities of superoxide dismutase (SOD) and glutathione peroxidase were lower in patients with Alzheimer's disease as well as in elderly subjects with mild cognitive impairment compared to those of normal individuals (Rinaldi et al. 2003). In another study plasma vitamin C levels were lower in subjects with dementia than in normal individuals (Charlton et al. 2004).

These studies suggest that lower levels of antioxidants in the body may contribute to increased oxidative stress, which initiates the development of Alzheimer's disease and participates in its progression.

Human Studies with Melatonin

Patients with Alzheimer's disease often exhibit both agitated behavior and poor sleep patterns. In a clinical study supplementation with melatonin failed to affect these abnormal symptoms in Alzheimer's patients compared to a placebo group (Gehrman et al. 2009).

However, melatonin in combination with standard therapy produced beneficial effects on cognitive function and depression more than that produced by standard therapy alone (Furio, Brusco, and Cardinali 2007).

Thus, the effectiveness of melatonin alone in reducing abnormal behaviors in patients with Alzheimer's disease is not convincing.

Human Studies with NADH

It has been reported that the administration of NADH, a reduced form of NAD (nicotinamide adenine dehydrogenase; 10 milligrams per day) improved cognitive function in Alzheimer's patients (Birkmayer 1996).

This observation was not confirmed by another clinical study in which supplementation with NADH produced no effect in improving cognitive function in patients with mild to moderate Alzheimer's (Rainer et al. 2000).

Human Studies with Omega-3 Fatty Acids

In a clinical study of patients with mild to moderate Alzheimer's, supplementation with omega-3 fatty acids (1.7 grams of docosahexaenoic acid and 0.6 g of eicosapentaenoic acid) did not delay the rate of cognitive decline. However, beneficial effects were observed in a small group of patients with very mild Alzheimer's disease (Freund-Levi et al. 2006).

A review of several survey-types of studies and clinical trials suggest that omega-3 fatty acids may slow down cognitive decline in elderly individuals without dementia, but it was ineffective in reducing the incidence of Alzheimer's or dementia (Fotuhi, Mohassel, and Yaffe 2009).

In the Canadian Study of Health and Aging (CSHA), there was no association between omega-3 fatty acids and the risk of developing dementia (Kroger et al. 2009). In another clinical study supplementation with omega-3 fatty acids showed significant improvement in the Alzheimer's Disease Assessment Scale (ADAS-cog) in individuals with mild cognitive impairment compared to those individuals who received no omega-3 fatty acids (placebo control). However, there was no significant difference in patients with Alzheimer's disease compared to the placebo group (Chiu et al. 2008).

These studies suggest that treatment with omega-3 fatty acids alone does not produce consistent beneficial effects in patients with Alzheimer's.

Human Studies with Resveratrol

Several survey-type studies suggest that the moderate consumption of red wine is associated with a lower incidence of Alzheimer's disease and dementia in the general population, and the consumption of three servings of wine daily was associated with a lower risk of Alzheimer's in elderly individuals without the APOE 4-allele (Luchsinger et al. 2004).

CONCLUDING REMARKS

Many research studies have been undertaken in order to attempt to reduce the incidence and progression of Alzheimer's disease. These studies have identified some important biochemical and genetic defects that manifest with the disease. We have identified that increased oxidative stress initiates the development of Alzheimer's disease, while other biochemical defects, such as increased chronic inflammation, mitochondrial dysfunction, beta-amyloids, and protesome inhibition occur subsequent to increased oxidative stress.

The genetic defects in certain genes (mutations in amyloid precursor protein or APP, presenilin-1, and presenilin-2 genes) are found in familial Alzheimer's disease. These mutations increase the production of beta-amyloids that cause degeneration of the nerve cells via free radicals. Increased oxidative stress together with these other biochemical and genetic defects participate in the progression of Alzheimer's disease.

Laboratory studies show that treatment with individual dietary antioxidants, endogenous antioxidants, B vitamins, omega-3 fatty acids, and certain polyphenolic compounds protected nerve cells and improved some symptoms in animal Alzheimer's models. A few clinical studies with an individual antioxidant have produced inconsistent results in patients with mild to moderate Alzheimer's. This is to be expected, however, given that the use of one or two antioxidants is unlikely to increase the levels of antioxidant enzymes and dietary and endogenous antioxidants.

I suggest that reducing oxidative stress and chronic inflammation by agents that can increase the levels of antioxidant enzymes as well as dietary and endogenous antioxidant chemicals at the same time may be one of the most effective ways to reduce the incidence of Alzheimer's disease in high-risk populations.

In the following chapter I provide specific recommendations as to how this could and should be done.

7 Alzheimer's Disease Prevention and Management

Micronutrients, Diet, and Lifestyle Recommendations

At present the treatment of Alzheimer's disease remains totally unsatisfactory. This is due in part to the fact that the drugs used for its treatment are meant to cure the symptoms of the disease instead of targeting its cause. None of the drugs currently employed have had any significant effect on the contributing factors of increased oxidative stress and chronic inflammation; therefore, neurons continue to die. *Increasing* the levels of antioxidant defense systems (antioxidant enzymes and dietary and endogenous antioxidants) as an adjunct to standard therapy may reduce the progression—as well as improve the symptoms—of Alzheimer's disease more than that produced by standard therapy alone.

As we know the use of one or two antioxidants is unlikely to achieve the aforementioned goal of optimally reducing oxidative stress and chronic inflammation. In order to reduce oxidative stress and chronic inflammation optimally, it's essential to use a combination of agents that can both increase the levels of antioxidant enzymes through the activation of nuclear transcriptional factor Nrf2, as well as increase

109

the levels of dietary and endogenous antioxidant chemicals in the body. Laboratory studies show that treatment with individual dietary antioxidants, endogenous antioxidants, B vitamins, omega-3 fatty acids, and certain polyphenolic compounds protects nerve cells and improves some symptoms in animal Alzheimer's models.

This chapter briefly describes rationales for using a preparation of micronutrients containing multiple dietary and endogenous antioxidants as well as certain polyphenolic compounds and aspirin for the primary prevention of Alzheimer's disease. The same proposed formulation of micronutrients and aspirin can be used in secondary prevention, and in combination with standard therapy, for the improved management of Alzheimer's disease in humans.

This preparation should be tested by clinical studies, but may also be utilized by populations that are at a high risk for developing Alzheimer's disease in consultation with their physicians. It is found in Table 7.1.

THE PROBLEM OF USING
A SINGLE NUTRIENT
TO TREAT ALZHEIMER'S DISEASE

Several studies showed the beneficial effects of single antioxidants, B vitamins, omega-3 fatty acids, and certain polyphenolic compounds alone in animal and cell-culture models of Alzheimer's. However, supplements with these individual agents did not produce the anticipated beneficial effects in high-risk human populations or in patients with mild to moderate forms of the disease.

As we have established elsewhere in this book but bears repeating here, individuals afflicted with a chronic disease such as Alzheimer's have an elevated internal oxidative environment. This suggests that the administration of a single antioxidant would result in oxidation of the administered antioxidant. Because an oxidized antioxidant acts as a pro-oxidant (like a free radical) it may not produce beneficial clinical outcomes. Indeed, a few clinical studies with an individual antioxidant failed to produce the beneficial effects in humans that were observed in animal models. The reality is, in fact, that an oxidized antioxidant is likely to *increase one's risk of developing Alzheimer's disease* after long-term consumption.

This same conclusion regarding the effects of a single antioxidant has also been shown to apply to previous studies of chronic diseases other than Alzheimer's. One such study involved beta-carotene in heavy male smokers for reducing the risk of lung cancer. The results of this study showed harmful effects to these smokers (Albanes et al. 1995).

Another study involved vitamin E and Parkinson's disease. The results of that study showed that vitamin E had no effect on the disease (Shoulson 1998).

THE RATIONALE FOR USING MULTIPLE ANTIOXIDANTS IN THE TREATMENT OF ALZHEIMER'S DISEASE

When one understands the complexities of how antioxidants function in the human body, one is able to comprehend why it's necessary to use a variety of them to reduce the risk and improve the management of Alzheimer's disease. The mechanisms of action of antioxidants vary greatly: their distribution in various organs and cells, their affinity to various types of free radicals, and their biological half-lives are all different. For example, beta-carotene is more effective in scavenging oxygen radicals than most of the other antioxidants. Beta-carotene can perform certain biological functions that cannot be performed by vitamin A, and Vitamin A can perform certain biological functions that cannot be performed by beta-carotene.

It has been reported that beta-carotene treatment enhances the expression of the connexin gene, which codes for a gap junction protein in mammalian fibroblasts in culture (Zhang et al. 1992). Vitamin A treatment doesn't produce such an effect. Vitamin A can induce differentiation in certain normal and cancer cells, whereas beta-carotene and other carotenoids cannot. Thus, beta-carotene and vitamin A, to some extent, have different functions in the body.

The gradient of oxygen pressure varies within the cells of the human body. Some antioxidants such as vitamin E are more effective as scavengers of free radicals in an environment marked by reduced oxygen pressure, whereas beta-carotene and vitamin A are more effective in environments that are characterized by higher atmospheric pressure.

Cells contain mostly water and some fat. Cellular components are distributed in the water and fat of the cells. Vitamin C is necessary to protect cellular components in the water portion of the cells, whereas vitamin A, carotenoids, and vitamin E protect cellular components in the fat portion of the cells. Vitamin C also plays an important role in maintaining cellular levels of vitamin E by recycling the oxidized form of vitamin E (wherein it acts as a pro-oxidant) to the reduced form of vitamin E (wherein it acts as an antioxidant).

The *form* of vitamin E used in a micronutrient preparation is also very important. It has been established that d-alpha-tocopheryl succinate (vitamin E succinate) is the most effective form of vitamin E both *in vitro* and *in vivo*. This form of vitamin E is more soluble than alpha-tocopherol and enters cells more readily. Therefore, it's expected to cross the blood-brain barrier in greater amounts than alpha-tocopherol.

We've reported that an oral ingestion of alpha-tocopheryl succinate (800 IU per day) in humans increased the plasma levels not only of alpha-tocopherol, but also vitamin E succinate. This suggests that a portion of vitamin E succinate can be absorbed from the intestinal tract before conversion to alpha-tocopherol. This observation is important because the conventional assumption based on the studies in rodents has been that esterified forms of vitamin E, such as alpha-tocopheryl succinate, alpha-tocopheryl nicotinate, and alpha-tocopheryl acetate, can be absorbed from the intestinal tract only *after* they are converted to the alpha-tocopherol form. Again, our preliminary data showed that this assumption may not be true for the absorption of vitamin E succinate in humans, provided the pool of alpha-tocopherol in the blood is saturated.

The endogenous antioxidant glutathione is effective in destroying H_2O_2 and superoxide anion (a form of free radical). However, oral supplementation with glutathione failed to significantly increase the plasma levels of glutathione in humans, suggesting that glutathione is completely destroyed in the intestine. Therefore, I propose to utilize N-acetylcysteine (NAC) and alpha-lipoic acid, which increase the cellular levels of glutathione by different mechanisms in a micronutrient preparation.

Another endogenous antioxidant, coenzyme Q10, may have some potential value in the prevention and improved treatment of Alzheimer's disease. Coenzyme Q10 administration has been shown to improve clinical symptoms in patients with mitochondrial encephalomyopathies (Chen, Huang, and Chu 1997). Due to the fact that mitochondrial dysfunction is associated with Alzheimer's and because coenzyme Q10 is needed for the generation of ATP by mitochondria, it is essential to add this antioxidant to a micronutrient preparation. A study has shown that coenzyme Q10 scavenges peroxy radicals faster than alpha-tocopherol, and like vitamin C, can convert oxidized vitamin E to the reduced form of vitamin E, which acts as an antioxidant (Niki 1997 and Hiramatsu et al 1991).

Glutamate may be involved in inducing fear and anxiety in patients with Alzheimer's. Nicotinamide (vitamin B_3) attenuated glutamate-induced toxicity in nerve cells. Nicotinamide is also an inhibitor of histone deacetylase activity and has restored memory deficits in Alzheimer's transgenic mice. These preclinical data suggest that oral supplementation with nicotinamide may be safe and useful in the prevention and improved treatment of Alzheimer's disease. Selenium is a cofactor of glutathione peroxidase, and Se-glutathione peroxidase acts as an antioxidant by increasing the intracellular level of glutathione.

In addition to dietary and endogenous antioxidants, B vitamins— and especially high doses of vitamin B_3 (nicotinamide)—should be added to our multiple micronutrient preparation. B vitamins are essential for normal brain function. Omega-3 fatty acids are also added because most clinical studies show some benefits of their inclusion in patients with Alzheimer's disease.

Two recent clinical studies showed that supplementation with multivitamin preparations reduced cancer incidence by 10 percent in men (Gaziano et al. 2012) and improved clinical outcomes in patients with HIV/AIDS who were not taking medication (Baum et al. 2013).

THE RATIONALE FOR USING A LOW-DOSE NSAID IN ALZHEIMER'S DISEASE PREVENTION

Since inflammatory reactions represent one of the major defects that participate in the development and progression of Alzheimer's, the use of nonsteroidal anti-inflammatory drugs (NSAIDs) appears to be a rational choice for the prevention and improved management of Alzheimer's. Laboratory, epidemiological (survey-type study), and clinical studies support this. Laboratory data have shown that products of inflammatory reactions, such as prostaglandins (Prasad et al. 1998), cytokines (Shalit et al. 1994; Sharif et al. 1993), complement proteins (Rogers et al. 1995; Webster, O'Barr, and Rogers 1994), adhesion molecules (Rozemuller et al. 1989; Verbeek et al. 1994), and free radicals (Harman 1992; Smith et al. 1995), are toxic to nerve cells.

Survey-type studies have revealed that rheumatoid arthritis patients on high doses of nonsteroidal anti-inflammatory drugs (NSAIDs) had a reduced incidence of Alzheimer's disease (Breitner et al. 1994; Andersen et al. 1995; McGeer and McGeer 1998).

NSAIDs also decreased the rate of deterioration of cognitive functions in Alzheimer's patients (Brown et al. 2000; Lucca et al. 1994; Rogers et al. 1993). However, the administration of prednisone, a powerful anti-inflammatory agent, was not useful in patients with Alzheimer's disease (Aisen et al. 2000).

In another survey-type study it was found that the use of NSAIDs and salicylates that did not contain barbiturates was associated with a lower risk of developing Alzheimer's disease and dementia when compared to all other causative factors (Cote et al. 2012).

Treatment with a mixed cyclooxygenase-1 (COX-1/COX-2 inhibitors) and a prostaglandin E2 (PGE2) analog failed to produce any significant benefit on cognitive function in patients with Alzheimer's (Scharf et al. 1999). A specific inhibitor of COX-2 was also not useful in improving cognitive function in patients with Alzheimer's disease (Sainati, Ingram, and Talwalker 2000). Therefore, it was suggested that the COX-2 enzyme may not be the appropriate target for Alzheimer's disease treatment (McGeer 2000).

In contrast to the COX-2 inhibitor, treatment with the selective COX-1 inhibitor SC-560 improved spatial learning and memory and decreased beta-amyloid deposits and tau hyperphosphorylation in old, triple transgenic Alzheimer's mice (3xTg). In addition, treatment with SC-560 reduced glial activation and markers of chronic inflammation (Choi et al. 2013).

Administration of indomethacin-loaded lipid-core nanocapsules blocked beta-amyloid-induced inflammation and suppressed glial and microglia activation (Bernardi et al. 2012).

Treatment of human neuronal cells in culture with both vitamin C and aspirin inhibited inflammatory responses more than that by aspirin alone (Candelario-Jalil et al. 2006).

The potential value of NSAIDs is supported by some additional studies. For example, the brains of nondemented elderly people taking NSAIDs had fewer activated microglia, suggesting reduced anti-inflammatory activity (Mackenzie and Munoz 1998).

Chronic administration of ibuprofen reduced inflammation and beta-amyloid deposition in the brain of a transgenic animal Alzheimer's model (Lim et al. 2000). Thus, the use of NSAIDs as a preventive agent of Alzheimer's disease remains a viable option.

CAN FAMILIAL ALZHEIMER'S DISEASE BE PREVENTED OR DELAYED?

It is often believed that the familial Alzheimer's disease (a family history of Alzheimer's) cannot be prevented or delayed by any pharmacological and/or physiological means. However, laboratory experiments on the genetic basis of another disease model (cancer) in *Drosophila melanogaster* (fruit fly) show that it may be possible to prevent or at least delay the onset of the familial basis of Alzheimer's.

The gene HOP (TUM-1) is essential for the development of fruit flies. A mutation in this gene markedly increases the risk of developing a leukemia-like tumor in female flies (unpublished observation in collaboration with Dr. Bhattacharya et al. of NASA, Moffat Field, California). Proton radiation is a powerful cancer-causing agent. Whole-body irradiation with proton radiation dramatically increased the incidence of cancer in these irradiated flies compared to that in unirradiated flies.

The question arose as to whether or not a preparation of multiple antioxidants can reduce the incidence of cancer that occurs as a result of a specific gene defect. To test this possibility a mixture of multiple dietary and endogenous antioxidants were fed to these flies via the diet seven days before proton irradiation and continued throughout the experimental period of seven days. The results showed that antioxidant treatment before and after irradiation totally blocked the proton radiation-induced cancer in fruit flies. This finding on fruit flies is of particular interest because to my knowledge this is the first demonstration in which the genetic basis of a disease can be prevented by supplementation with multiple antioxidants. This observation made on fruit flies cannot readily be extrapolated to humans.

Specifically, regarding the children of parents who have a family history of Alzheimer's, it's not known whether Alzheimer's disease can be prevented or delayed in them by giving them a daily supplementation of multiple antioxidants. The results with fruit flies suggest that it could. A clinical study to test the effectiveness of the proposed strategies among those who have a family history of Alzheimer's should be conducted.

PRIMARY AND SECONDARY PREVENTION STRATEGIES

The purpose of primary prevention is to protect healthy individuals from developing Alzheimer's, while the purpose of secondary prevention is to stop or slow the progression of risk factors in those individuals who are at a high risk of developing Alzheimer's disease. As has been established these high-risk individuals include people age sixty-five and older and those with a family history of the disease.

The strategies proposed for primary prevention may also be used for secondary prevention in individuals with early phase Alzheimer's disease who are not taking any medication.

Primary Prevention

In order to develop primary prevention strategies, it's essential to identify external risk factors that increase the risk of developing Alzheimer's disease. Some human epidemiologic and animal studies have identified environment-, diet-, and lifestyle-related risk factors that impact here. As discussed in chapter 3, agents that may *increase* the risk of Alzheimer's include the high consumption of aluminum from drinking water (Rondeau et al. 2009), a high-fat/high-cholesterol diet (Thirumangalakudi et al. 2008), a vitamin D deficiency (Evatt et al. 2008), cigarette smoking (Ho et al. 2012), exposure to electromagnetic fields (Jiang et al. 2013), and exposure to chronic noise (Cui et al. 2012). Although there are no conclusive data on the degree to which these external risk factors may increase the risk of Alzheimer's disease in humans, I would suggest that exposure to these factors should be minimized for its primary prevention.

Exercise may reduce the risk of developing Alzheimer's (Souza et al. 2013). In addition, daily mental exercise may be beneficial in this regard. It has been reported that a high dietary intake of vitamin C and vitamin E may also reduce the risk of developing Alzheimer's.

Among current cigarette smokers, the intake of beta-carotene and flavonoids may decrease the risk of Alzheimer's disease (Engelhart et al. 2002). Although there are no conclusive data on the effectiveness of these external risk factors in reducing the risk of Alzheimer's in humans, I would suggest that adopting exercise and maintaining a sufficient intake of dietary antioxidants would be a good approach for its primary prevention.

Any studies done as regards primary prevention should target individuals with a family history of Alzheimer's who have not developed any symptoms of the disease and those age sixty-five or older.

Secondary Prevention

Let's now take a look at secondary prevention strategies, which attempt to influence the risk factors involved in the development of the disease and improve its symptoms. Individuals who exhibit early signs of Alzheimer's but are not taking any medication may be included in secondary prevention. External risk factors that increase the risk of developing Alzheimer's disease are the same as they are for primary prevention, as stated above: the high consumption of aluminum from drinking water, a high-fat/high-cholesterol diet, a vitamin D deficiency, cigarette smoking, exposure to electromagnetic fields, and exposure to chronic noise.

Internal risk factors include increased oxidative stress, mitochondrial dysfunction, chronic inflammation, increased production of beta-amyloids from APP, inhibition of proteasome activity, and high cholesterol levels. Beta-amyloids cause damage to the nerve cells by producing free radicals. Thus, reducing exposure to external risk factors and internal biochemical defects may be one of the rational options for secondary prevention.

Any studies done as regards secondary prevention should target individuals with an early phase of Alzheimer's disease.

SUGGESTED MICRONUTRIENTS

In designing an optimal study of Alzheimer's, or for individuals at high risk for developing Alzheimer's disease, the ingredients for consumption are of paramount importance. The select combination of non-toxic agents that should be included are vitamin A (retinyl palmitate), B vitamins with higher levels of vitamin B_3 (nicotinamide), vitamin C (calcium ascorbate), vitamin D, vitamin E (both d-alpha-tocopheryl acetate and d-alpha-tocopheryl succinate), natural mixed carotenoids, selenium, coenzyme Q10, alpha-lipoic acid, N-acetylcysteine (NAC), L-carnitine, omega-3 fatty acids, resveratrol, curcumin, and a low-dose aspirin.

This particular combination of agents was selected because they are capable of optimally reducing oxidative stress and chronic inflammation by enhancing the levels of antioxidant enzymes through the activation of the Nrf2 by ROS-independent mechanism and by enhancing the levels of antioxidant chemicals that directly scavenge free radicals. Again, the doses of all of these ingredients are listed in Table 7.1. In addition to suggesting that these ingredients be utilized in studies to be undertaken, they are also suggested for populations at high risk for the development of Alzheimer's or for those individuals with dementia, with or without Alzheimer's disease. This preparation, called "Brain-Seva," is commercially available from Randal Optimal Nutrients, www.randaloptimal.com.

The following dose amounts are for adults. For children age five to twelve, with a family history of Alzheimer's, the dose should be 20 percent of the adult dose. For adolescents age thirteen to seventeen, also with a family history of Alzheimer's, the dose should be 40 percent of the adult dose. These ingredients are best taken half in the morning, half in the evening, both times with a meal.

TABLE 7.1. INGREDIENTS OF A RECOMMENDED MICRONUTRIENT PREPARATION FOR HIGH-RISK POPULATIONS AND PATIENTS WITH DEMENTIA WITH OR WITHOUT ALZHEIMER'S DISEASE (DAILY DOSES)

Vitamin A (retinal palmitate)	3,000 IU
Vitamin B$_1$ (thiamine mononitrate)	10 mg
Vitamin B$_2$ (riboflavin)	4 mg
Vitamin B$_3$ (nicotinamide)	100 mg
Vitamin B$_6$ (pyridoxine hydrochloride)	4 mg
Vitamin B$_7$ (biotin)	150 mcg
Vitamin B$_9$ (folic acid)	400 mcg
Vitamin B$_{12}$ (Methyl cobalamin)	1,000 mcg
Vitamin C (calcium ascorbate)	1,000 mg
Vitamin D$_3$ (cholecalciferol)	1,000 IU
Natural Vitamin E	400 IU (d-alpha-tocopheryl succinate–250 IU) (d-alpha-tocopheryl acetate–150 IU)
Pantothenic Acid (D-calcium pantothenate)	15 mg
Selenium (seleno-L-methionine)	100 mcg
Zinc Glycinate	5 mg
Coenzyme Q10	proprietary dose*
Curcumin	proprietary dose
L-carnitine	proprietary dose
N-acetylcysteine (NAC)	proprietary dose
Omega-3 fatty acids	proprietary dose
R-alpha-lipoic acid	proprietary dose
Trans-resveratrol	proprietary dose
Mixed carotenoids	proprietary dose

*Total amount of antioxidants in herbal products is 1,585 mg

Toxicity Concerns and Considerations

Antioxidants, B vitamins, and certain polyphenolic compounds (curcumin and resveratrol) used in the proposed micronutrient preparation are considered safe. Antioxidants at doses higher than those that are recommended for the proposed micronutrient preparation have been consumed by the U.S. population for decades without significant toxicity. However, a few of the ingredients could produce harmful effects at certain high doses in some individuals when consumed daily for a long period of time.

For example, vitamin A at doses of 10,000 IU or more per day can cause birth defects in pregnant women, and beta-carotene at doses of 50 milligrams or more can produce bronzing of the skin that is reversible on discontinuation. Vitamin C as ascorbic acid at high doses (10 grams or more per day) can cause diarrhea in some individuals. Vitamin E at high doses (2,000 IU or more per day) can induce clotting defects after long-term consumption. Vitamin B_6 at high doses (50 milligrams or more per day) may produce peripheral neuropathy, and selenium at doses 400 micrograms or more per day can cause skin and liver toxicity after long-term consumption. Coenzyme Q10 has no known toxicity; recommended daily doses are 30 to 400 milligrams. N-acetylcysteine (NAC) at doses of 250 to 1,500 milligrams and alpha-lipoic acid at doses of 600 milligrams are used in humans without toxicity. All ingredients present in the proposed micronutrient preparations are safe. They are categorized as "Food Supplement" and therefore do not require FDA approval for their use.

The proposed formulation of micronutrients has no iron, copper, manganese, or heavy metals (vanadium, zirconium, and molybdenum). Iron and copper aren't added because they're known to interact with vitamin C and generate excessive amounts of free radicals. In addition, iron and copper are absorbed more in the presence of antioxidants than in their absence. Therefore, it's possible that prolonged consumption of these trace minerals in the presence of antioxidants may increase the levels of free iron or copper stores in the body, because there are no significant mechanisms of iron excretion among postmenopausal women and men of all ages. Increased stores of free iron or copper may increase the risk of some chronic human diseases, including Alzheimer's disease. High levels of these metals are considered neurotoxic.

The effectiveness of the proposed micronutrient preparation and low-dose aspirin on high-risk populations should be tested by a well-designed clinical study.

THE INCLUSION OF ASPIRIN

Low-dose aspirin is recommended for inclusion in the formula to be used by adults because of its anti-inflammatory effect and because in combination with vitamin E, it produced a synergistic effect on the inhibition of cyclooxygenase activity (Abate et al. 2000). Therefore, the combination of aspirin and vitamin E may be more effective in reducing levels of chronic inflammation than the individual agents.

Indeed, consumption of vitamin C and vitamin E in combination with NSAIDs was associated with reduced cognitive decline over time in elderly individuals with an APOE-epsilon-4-allele (Fotuhi et al. 2008). A low-dose aspirin (81 milligrams per day) is recommended by cardiologists to reduce the risk of heart disease; however, it can cause intestinal bleeding in some individuals after long-term consumption.

RECOMMENDED DOSE SCHEDULE

Most clinical Alzheimer's studies with antioxidants have utilized a once-a-day dose-schedule. As we have previously established, taking vitamins and antioxidants once a day can create large fluctuations of their levels in the body. This is due to the fact that the biological half-lives of vitamins and antioxidants markedly vary depending on their lipid or water solubility. A two-fold difference in the levels of vitamin

E succinate can produce marked alterations in the expression profiles of several genes in nerve cells in culture. Therefore, taking a multivitamin preparation once a day may produce a large fluctuation in the levels of micronutrients in the body, which could potentially cause genetic stress in the cells. This stress may compromise the effectiveness of the vitamin supplementation after long-term consumption.

I recommend taking the proposed preparation of micronutrients twice a day in order to improve its effectiveness and to reduce fluctuations in the levels of gene expression in the body. The daily doses can be divided in two (half taken in the morning and half in the evening, preferably with a meal at both times).

CURRENT TREATMENTS OF ALZHEIMER'S DISEASE

The purpose of treatment is to improve the symptoms and reduce the progression of the disease. However, treatment protocols for Alzheimer's disease today, while improving some of its symptoms, have failed to stop the progression of the disease. Drugs that are commonly prescribed for Alzheimer's include cholinesterase inhibitors (donepezil, galantamine, and rivastigmine), and the N-methyl-D-aspartate (NMDA) antagonist (memantine).

The purpose of cholinesterase inhibitors is to improve cognitive function by increasing the acetylcholine levels in cholinergic neurons. The beneficial effects of these drugs depend upon the viability of surviving cholinergic neurons. The purpose of the NMDA receptor antagonist is to stop the action of glutamate, which induces fear and anxiety in patients with Alzheimer's. In randomized, double-blind, placebo-controlled clinical trials, all acetylcholinesterase inhibitors (AChEIs) have shown varying degrees of effectiveness in improving cognitive function in patients with mild to moderate Alzheimer's disease. No such improvement was observed in the placebo group who did not receive the drug.

When comparing donepezil, galantamine, and rivastigmine, donepezil was found to be slightly more effective than the other drugs (Lopez-Pousa et al. 2005). However, other researchers have reported no such difference between these drugs (Birks and Flicker 2006).

In Hispanic populations the safety and beneficial effects of donepezil on cognitive function were similar to those found in the general population (Lopez et al. 2008). The annual cost of donepezil, galantamine, and rivastigmine was not significantly different (Mucha et al. 2008).

Statins are commonly used in the prevention and treatment of heart disease. Treatment with the statins atorvastatin and pitavastatin reduced senile plaques and the inflammation marker TNF-alpha in the transgenic Alzheimer's model (App-Tg) mice by reducing oxidative stress and improving insulin signaling pathways (Kurata et al. 2013). The efficacy of these statins in human Alzheimer's disease has not been tested.

Using old transgenic Alzheimer's mice model (APP/swePS1 Δ E9), it was shown that oral administration of the memory-enhancing neurotrophic molecule J147 improved cognitive function even when administered at a late stage of the disease (Prior et al. 2013). This effect of J147 is mediated by inducing NGF and several BDNF-responsive proteins, which are considered important for learning and memory. The efficacy of these growth factors in human Alzheimer's has not been tested.

LIMITATIONS OF CURRENT MEDICATIONS IN TREATING ALZHEIMER'S DISEASE

It has been proposed that the gradual loss of cognitive functions in Alzheimer's is due to the loss of cholinergic neurons. Therefore, cholinergic drugs (acetylcholinesterase inhibitors) are used to improve the function of surviving neurons in Alzheimer's patients. However, these agents do not protect cholinergic neurons from the damaging effects of free radicals and the products of chronic inflammation. Consequently, the nerve cells die off and the beneficial effects of cholinergic drugs do not last long.

RECOMMENDED MICRONUTRIENTS AND A LOW-DOSE ASPIRIN IN COMBINATION WITH STANDARD THERAPY IN PATIENTS WITH DEMENTIA WITH OR WITHOUT ALZHEIMER'S DISEASE

The presence of senile plaques and NFTs in the brain is characteristic of Alzheimer's disease; they are absent in patients with age-related dementia. It has been observed that the gradual loss of cognitive functions in patients with Alzheimer's as well as in patients with dementia without the presence of senile plaques and neurofibrillary tangles (NFTs) is due to the progressive loss of cholinergic neurons from the brain. Some viable cholinergic neurons are present in the brain in patients with mild to moderate Alzheimer's and in age-related dementia.

Drugs that inhibit acetylcholinesterase activity are used to improve cognitive function by enhancing the levels of acetylcholine in surviving cholinergic neurons in Alzheimer's patients. It is essential that cholinergic neurons are viable in order for the drug to produce beneficial effects on cognitive functions. However, these drugs do not protect cholinergic neurons from the damaging effects of free radicals and chronic inflammation, and thus they die.

The beneficial effects of drugs last as long as neurons are alive. As mentioned earlier supplementation with an antagonist of glutamate receptor NMDA can be useful in reducing anxiety and fear in Alzheimer's patients. This drug also does not affect oxidative stress or chronic inflammation. Antioxidants reduce the release and toxicity of glutamate on the nerve cells in the brain. Aspirin enhances the anti-inflammatory effects of antioxidants. Therefore, an addition of the micronutrient preparation and a low-dose aspirin in combination with standard therapy may prolong the beneficial effects of current drugs in patients with Alzheimer's disease as well as in patients with age-related dementia by protecting surviving neurons from the damaging effects of free radicals, chronic inflammation, and glutamate.

DIET AND LIFESTYLE RECOMMENDATIONS FOR ALZHEIMER'S

Even though there's no direct link between environment-, diet-, and lifestyle-related factors and the initiation and progression of Alzheimer's, it would be beneficial to avoid exposure to aluminum, as well as an excess consumption of iron, copper, manganese, and zinc. Dietary recommendations include a balanced diet that is high in fiber and low in fat, with plenty of fruits and vegetables. A low-calorie diet appears to be useful in improving memory. Among the fruits blueberries and raspberries are particularly important because of their protective role against oxidative injuries in the brain. Lifestyle recommendations include moderate exercise daily, reduced stress, no tobacco smoking, and reduced exposure to noise and electromagnetic pulses.

CONCLUDING REMARKS

It is proposed that a combination of agents—which can simultaneously increase the levels of antioxidant enzymes through the activation of Nrf2 by a ROS-independent mechanism and antioxidant chemicals which can directly scavenge free radicals—may be necessary to reduce oxidative stress optimally to inhibit the development and progression of Alzheimer's disease and, in combination with standard medication, may improve the management of this disease. Dietary and endogenous antioxidants, vitamin D, B vitamins with higher doses of vitamin B_3, curcumin, resveratrol, and omega-3 fatty acids can fulfill the above-mentioned requirements for reducing oxidative stress and chronic inflammation optimally.

A low-dose nonsteroidal anti-inflammatory drug (NSAID) such as aspirin (81 milligrams per day) is recommended only for the adults who have early phase Alzheimer's disease or have established dementia with or without Alzheimer's disease. This preparation of micronutrients would also protect against glutamate-induced fear and anxiety, as well as damage to the nerve cells. All ingredients in the proposed formulation are considered safe, which would allow their prolonged usage in those individuals who are at high risk of developing Alzheimer's. The suggested dose-schedule of twice a day would reduce fluctuations in the levels of vitamins and antioxidants that can impact gene expression in the cells. Clinical studies using the proposed recommendations for primary and secondary prevention should also be initiated.

Current drug treatments are based on the symptoms rather than the causes of Alzheimer's disease. Standard therapy has produced transient benefits on some symptoms such as improving cognitive function. However, the drugs used in standard therapy don't have any effect on the increased oxidative stress and chronic inflammation that are responsible for neuronal degeneration. Consequently, the neurons of the afflicted individual continue to die, despite an adherence to medication on the part of the afflicted individual.

The effectiveness of cholinesterase inhibitors in improving cognitive function lasts as long as the cholinergic neurons are viable. The currently used drugs have severe side effects. The strategies recommended for primary prevention can also be used in combination with standard medications to improve the management of Alzheimer's by reducing the progression of the disease and prolonging the effectiveness of the drugs on cognitive functions.

Again, dietary recommendations include a low-fat, high-fiber diet with plenty of fruits and vegetables and the reduced consumption of iron, copper, aluminum, and zinc. Lifestyle recommendations include daily moderate exercise, reducing stress, the cessation of tobacco smoking, and the reduced exposure to noise and the electromagnetic field. Clinical studies using the proposed recommendations in combination with standard therapy for the improved management of Alzheimer's disease should be initiated. In the meantime those interested in the proposed micronutrient approach in prevention or for the improved management of Alzheimer's or age-related dementia may like to adopt these recommendations in consultation with their physician or health care provider.

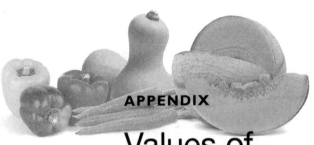

Values of Recommended Dietary Allowances (RDA)/ Dietary Reference Intakes (DRI)

Note to the Reader: All of the information contained in this appendix, including the tables, is from my book *Fighting Cancer with Vitamins and Antioxidants,* coauthored with my son K. C. Prasad, M.S., M.D., published by Healing Arts Press in 2011.

■ ■ ■

Sufficient changes in nutritional guidelines have occurred since World War II due to our increased knowledge of nutrition and health. The nutritional guidelines referred to as Recommended Dietary Allowances (RDAs) were first established in 1941. The Food and Nutrition Board of the United States subsequently revises these guidelines every five to ten years.

RDA (DRI)

RDA refers to the value of the daily dietary intake level of a nutrient considered sufficient to meet the requirements of 97 to 98 percent of healthy individuals of different ages and genders. Because of the rapid growth of research on the role of nutrients in human health, the Food and Nutrition Board of the Institute of Medicine (IOM) of the United States, in collaboration with Health Canada, updated the values of RDAs and renamed them Dietary Reference Intakes (DRIs) in 1998. Since then, DRI values are used by both countries. The DRI values of selected nutrients are listed in tables A.1 to A.21. The DRI values are not currently used in nutrition labeling; the RDA values of nutrients continue to be used for this purpose. The DRI values for carotenoids, alpha-lipoic acid, coenzyme Q10, and L-carnitine have not been determined.

ADEQUATE INTAKE (AI)

AI refers to the value of a nutrient for which no RDA has been established, but the value established may be sufficient for everyone in the demographic group.

TOLERABLE UPPER INTAKE LEVEL (UL)

The tolerable upper intake level is the maximum level of daily nutrient intake that is likely to pose no risk of adverse health effects. The UL value represents total intake of a nutrient from food, water, and supplements.

RELATIONSHIP BETWEEN RECOMMENDED DIETARY ALLOWANCE VALUES AND HEALTH

RDA values of nutrients are expected to be adequate for normal growth and survival; however, the values of micronutrients needed for prevention or improved management of human diseases are not known at this time. The data on doses obtained from the use of a single micronutrient in the prevention or treatment of Alzheimer's disease should not be extrapolated to the doses of the same micronutrient present in a multiple micronutrient preparation.

RDA/DRI values of micronutrients are sufficient for normal growth and survival, but they are not adequate for the prevention or improved treatment of human diseases. In order to evaluate the dosage of micronutrients in any multivitamin preparation for the prevention or improved treatment of Alzheimer's disease, it's essential to have sufficient knowledge of the RDA values of the micronutrients.

CONCLUDING REMARKS

The initial nutritional guidelines, Recommended Dietary Allowances (RDAs), have been replaced by Dietary Reference Intakes (DRIs) and are currently used in the United States and Canada. The DRI values of nutrients are sufficient for the growth and development of 97 to 98 percent of healthy individuals. The DRI values for carotenoids, alphalipoic acid, N-acetylcysteine, coenzyme Q10, and L-carnitine have not been determined. The optimal values needed for the prevention or improved management of Alzheimer's disease is not known. Both preventive and therapeutic doses of micronutrients are higher than their RDA values.

TABLE A.1. DIETARY REFERENCE
INTAKES (DRI) OF ANTIOXIDANT VITAMIN A

Age	RDA/AI*	UL
	µg/d (IU/d)	µg/d (IU/d)
Infants		
0–6 mo	400 (1,200 IU)*	600 (1,800 IU)
7–12 mo	500 (1,500 IU)*	600 (1,800 IU)
Children		
1–3 y	300 (900 IU)	600 (1,800 IU)
4–8 y	400 (1,200 IU)	900 (2,700 IU)
Males		
9–13 y	600 (1,800 IU)	1,700 (5,100 IU)
14–18 y	900 (2,700 IU)	2,800 (8,400 IU)
19 y and up	900 (2,700 IU)	3,000 (9,000 IU)
Females		
9–13 y	600 (1,800 IU)	1,700 (5,100 IU)
14–18 y	700 (2,100 IU)	2,800 (8,400 IU)
19 y and up	700 (2,100 IU)	3,000 (9,000 IU)
Pregnancy		
under 18 y	750 (2,250 IU)	2,800 (8,400 IU)
19–50 y	770 (2,310 IU)	3,000 (9,000 IU)
Lactation		
under 18 y	1,200 (3,600 IU)	2,800 (8,400 IU)
19–50 y	1,300 (3,900 IU)	3,000 (9,000 IU)

1 µg of retinol equals 1 µg of RAE (retinol activity equivalent); 1 IU of retinol equals 0.3 µg of retinol; and 2 µg of beta-carotene equals 1 µg of retinol.

RDA = Recommended Dietary Allowances
*AI = Adequate Intake
UL = Tolerable Upper Intake Value
µg = microgram; d = day

The values are adapted and summarized from the table of the Dietary Reference Intakes (DRI) published by www.nap.edu. (Search on "Food and Nutrition" and you will find information about DRI.)

TABLE A.2. DIETARY REFERENCE
INTAKES (DRI) OF ANTIOXIDANT VITAMIN C

Age	RDA/AI*	UL
	mg/d	mg/d
Infants		
0–6 mo	40*	ND
7–12 mo	50*	ND
Children		
1–3 y	15	400
4–8 y	25	650
Males		
9–13 y	45	1,200
14–18 y	75	1,800
19 y and up	90	2,000
Females		
9–13 y	45	1,200
14–18 y	65	1,800
19 y and up	75	2,000

RDA = Recommended Dietary Allowances
*AI = Adequate Intake
UL = Tolerable Upper Intake Value
µg = microgram; d = day

The values are adapted and summarized from the table of the Dietary Reference Intakes (DRI) published by www.nap.edu.

TABLE A.3. DIETARY REFERENCE
INTAKES (DRI) OF ANTIOXIDANT VITAMIN E

Age	RDA/AI*	UL
	mg/d (IU/d)	mg/d (IU/d)
Infants		
0–6 mo	4 (6 IU)*	ND
7–12 mo	5 (7.5 IU)*	ND
Children		
1–3 y	6 (9 IU)	200 (30 IU)
4–8 y	7 (10.6 IU)	300 (45 IU)
Males		
9–13 y	11 (16.7 IU)	600 (90 IU)
14–18 y	15 (22.8 IU)	800 (120 IU)
19 y and up	15 (22.8 IU)	1,000 (150 IU)
Females		
9–13 y	11 (16.7 IU)	600 (90 IU)
14–18 y	15 (22.8 IU)	800 (120 IU)
19 y and up	15 (22.8 IU)	1,000 (150 IU)
Pregnancy		
under 18 y	15 (22.8 IU)	800 (120 IU)
19–50 y	15 (22.8 IU)	1,000 (150 IU)
Lactation		
under 18 y	19 (28.9 IU)	800 (120 IU)
19–50 y	19 (28.9 IU)	1,000 (150 IU)

RDA = Recommended Dietary Allowances
*AI = Adequate Intake
UL = Tolerable Upper Intake Value
ND = not determined
mg = milligram; d = day
1 IU of vitamin E equals 0.66 mg of d- and 0.45 mg of
dl-alpha-tocopherol.

The values are adapted and summarized from the tables of the Dietary Reference Intakes (DRI)
published by www.nap.edu.

TABLE A.4. DIETARY REFERENCE
INTAKES (DRI) OF VITAMIN D

Age	RDA/AI*	UL
	µg/d (IU/d)	µg/d (IU/d)
Infants		
0–12 mo	5 (200 IU)*	25 (1,000 IU)
Children		
1–8 y	5 (200 IU)*	50 (2,000 IU)
Males		
9–50 y	5 (200 IU)*	50 (2,000 IU)
50–70 y	10 (400 IU)*	50 (2,000 IU)
over 70 y	15 (600 IU)*	50 (2,000 IU)
Females		
9–50 y	5 (200 IU)*	50 (2,000 IU)
50–70 y	10 (400 IU)*	50 (2,000 IU)
under 70 y	15 (600 IU)*	50 (2,000 IU)
Pregnancy		
18–50 y	5 (200 IU)*	50 (2,000 IU)
Lactation		
18–50 y	5 (200 IU)*	50 (2,000 IU)

RDA = Recommended Dietary Allowances
*AI = Adequate Intake
UL = Tolerable Upper Intake Value
µg = microgram; d = day
1 µg of cholecalciferol equals 40 IU (international unit)
of Vitamin D.

The values are adapted and summarized from the tables of the Dietary Reference Intakes (DRI)
published by www.nap.edu.

TABLE A.5. DIETARY REFERENCE
INTAKES (DRI) OF VITAMIN B₁ (THIAMINE)

Age	RDA/AI*	UL
	mg/d	mg/d
Infants		
0–6 mo	0.2*	ND
7–12 mo	0.3*	ND
Children		
1–3 y	0.5	ND
4–8 y	0.6	ND
Males		
9–13 y	0.9	ND
14 y and up	1.2	ND
Females		
9–13 y	0.9	ND
14–18 y	1.0	ND
19 y and up	1.1	ND
Pregnancy		
18–50 y	1.4	ND
Lactation		
18–50 y	1.4	ND

RDA = Recommended Dietary Allowances
*AI = Adequate Intake
UL = Tolerable Upper Intake Value
ND = not determined
mg = milligram; d = day

The values are adapted and summarized from the tables of the Dietary Reference Intakes (DRI) published by www.nap.edu.

TABLE A.6. DIETARY REFERENCE INTAKES (DRI) OF VITAMIN B₂ (RIBOFLAVIN)

Age	RDA/AI*	UL
	mg/d	mg/d
Infants		
0–6 mo	0.3*	ND
7–12 mo	0.4*	ND
Children		
1–3 y	0.5	ND
4–8 y	0.6	ND
Males		
9–13 y	0.9	ND
14 y and up	13	ND
Females		
9–13 y	0.9	ND
14–18 y	1.0	ND
19 y and up	1.1	ND
Pregnancy		
18–50 y	1.4	ND
Lactation		
18–50 y	1.6	ND

RDA = Recommended Dietary Allowances
*AI = Adequate Intake
UL = Tolerable Upper Intake Value
ND = not determined
mg = milligram; d = day

The values are adapted and summarized from the table of the Dietary Reference Intakes (DRI) published by www.nap.edu.

TABLE A.7. DIETARY REFERENCE
INTAKES (DRI) OF VITAMIN B$_6$

Age	RDA/AI*	UL
	mg/d	mg/d
Infants		
0–6 mo	0.1*	ND
7–12 mo	0.3*	ND
Children		
1–3 y	0.5	30
4–8 y	0.6	40
Males		
9–13 y	1.0	60
14–50 y	1.3	80
50–70 y and up	1.7	100
Females		
9–13 y	1.0	60
14–18 y	1.2	80
19–30 y	1.3	100
50 y and up	1.5	100
Pregnancy		
under 18 y	1.9	80
19–50 y	1.9	100
Lactation		
under 18 y	2.0	80
19–50 y	2.0	100

RDA = Recommended Dietary Allowances
*AI = Adequate Intake
UL = Tolerable Upper Intake Value
ND = not determined
mg = milligram; d = day

The values are adapted and summarized from the table of the Dietary Reference Intakes (DRI) published by www.nap.edu.

TABLE A.8. DIETARY REFERENCE INTAKES (DRI) OF VITAMIN B$_{12}$ (COBALAMIN)

Age	RDA/AI*	UL
	µg/d	µg/d
Infants		
0–6 mo	0.4*	ND
7–12 mo	0.5*	ND
Children		
1–3 y	0.9	ND
4–8 y	1.2	ND
Males		
9–13 y	1.08	ND
14 y and up	2.4	ND
Females		
9–13 y	1.8	ND
14 y and up	2.4	ND
Pregnancy		
18–50 y	2.6	ND
Lactation		
18–50 y	2.8	ND

RDA = Recommended Dietary Allowances
*AI = Adequate Intake
UL = Tolerable Upper Intake Value
ND = not determined
µg = microgram; d = day

The values are adapted and summarized from the table of the Dietary Reference Intakes (DRI) published by www.nap.edu.

TABLE A.9. DIETARY REFERENCE
INTAKES (DRI) OF VITAMIN PANTOTHENIC ACID

Age	RDA/AI*	UL
	mg/d	mg/d
Infants		
0–6 mo	1.7*	ND
7–12 mo	1.8*	ND
Children		
1–3 y	2*	ND
4–8 y	2*	ND
Males		
9–13 y	4*	ND
14 y and up	5*	ND
Females		
9–13 y	4*	ND
14 y and up	5*	ND
Pregnancy		
18–50 y	6*	ND
Lactation		
18–50 y	7*	ND

RDA = Recommended Dietary Allowances
*AI = Adequate Intake
UL = Tolerable Upper Intake Value
ND = not determined
mg = milligram; d = day

The values are adapted and summarized from the table of the Dietary Reference Intakes (DRI) published by www.nap.edu.

TABLE A.10. DIETARY REFERENCE INTAKES (DRI) OF VITAMIN NIACIN

Age	RDA/AI*	UL
	mg/d	mg/d
Infants		
0–6 mo	2*	ND
7–12 mo	0.4*	ND
Children		
1–3 y	6.0	10
4–8 y	8.0	15
Males		
9–13 y	12	20
14–50 y	16	30
50 y and up	16	35
Females		
9–13 y	12	20
14–18 y	14	30
19 y and up	14	35
Pregnancy		
under 18 y	18	30
19–50 y	18	35
Lactation		
under 18 y	17	30
19–50 y	17	35

RDA = Recommended Dietary Allowances
*AI = Adequate Intake
UL = Tolerable Upper Intake Value
ND = not determined
mg = milligram; d = day

The values are adapted and summarized from the table of the Dietary Reference Intakes (DRI) published by www.nap.edu

TABLE A.11. DIETARY REFERENCE
INTAKES (DRI) OF VITAMIN FOLATE

Age	RDA/AI*	UL
	µg/d	µg/d
Infants		
0–6 mo	65*	ND
7–12 mo	80*	ND
Children		
1–3 y	150	300
4–8 y	200	400
Males		
9–13 y	300	600
14–18 y	400	800
19 y and up	400	1,000
Females		
9–13 y	300	600
14–18 y	400	800
19 y and up	400	1,000
Pregnancy		
under 18 y	600	800
19–50 y	600	1,000
Lactation		
under 18 y	500	800
19–50 y	500	1,000

RDA = Recommended Dietary Allowances
*AI = Adequate Intake
UL = Tolerable Upper Intake Value
ND = not determined
µg = microgram; d = day

The values are adapted and summarized from the table of the Dietary Reference Intakes (DRI) published by www.nap.edu.

TABLE A.12. DIETARY REFERENCE INTAKES (DRI) OF MICRONUTRIENT BIOTIN

Age	RDA/AI*	UL
	µg/d	µg/d
Infants		
0–6 mo	0.5*	ND
7–12 mo	0.6*	ND
Children		
1–3 y	8*	ND
4–8 y	12*	ND
Males		
9–13 y	20	ND
14–18 y	25	ND
19 y and up	30	ND
Females		
9–13 y	20	ND
14–18 y	25	ND
19 y and up	30	ND
Pregnancy		
under 18 y	30*	ND
19–50 y	30*	ND
Lactation		
under 18 y	35*	ND
19–50 y	35*	ND

RDA = Recommended Dietary Allowances
*AI = Adequate Intake
UL = Tolerable Upper Intake Value
ND = not determined
µg = microgram; d = day

The values are adapted and summarized from the table of the Dietary Reference Intakes (DRI) published by www.nap.edu.

TABLE A.13. DIETARY REFERENCE
INTAKES (DRI) OF MINERAL CALCIUM

Age	RDA/AI*	UL
	mg/d	mg/d
Infants		
0–6 mo	210*	ND
7–12 mo	270*	ND
Children		
1–3 y	500*	2,500
4–8 y	800*	2,500
Males		
9–18 y	1,300*	2,500
19–50 y	1,000*	2,500
51 y and up	1,200*	2,500
Females		
9–8 y	1,300*	2,500
19–50 y	1,000*	2,500
51 y and up	1,200*	2,500
Pregnancy		
under 18 y	1,300*	2,500
19–50 y	1,000*	2,500
Lactation		
under 18 y	1,300*	2,500
19–50 y	1,000*	2,500

RDA = Recommended Dietary Allowances
*AI = Adequate Intake
UL = Tolerable Upper Intake Value
ND = not determined
mg = milligram; d = day

The values are adapted and summarized from the table of the Dietary Reference Intakes (DRI) published by www.nap.edu.

TABLE A.14. DIETARY REFERENCE INTAKES (DRI) OF MINERAL MAGNESIUM

Age	RDA/AI*	UL
	mg/d	mg/d
Infants		
0–6 mo	30*	ND
7–12 mo	75*	ND
Children		
1–3 y	80	65
4–8 y	130	110
Males		
9–13 y	240	350
14–18 y	410	350
19–30 y	400	350
31 y and up	420	350
Females		
9–13 y	240	350
14–18 y	360	350
31 y and up	320	350
Pregnancy		
under 18 y	400	350
19–30 y	350	350
31–50 y	360	350
Lactation		
under 18 y	360	350
31–50 y	320	350

RDA = Recommended Dietary Allowances
*AI = Adequate Intake
UL = Tolerable Upper Intake Value
ND = not determined
mg = milligram; d = day

The values are adapted and summarized from the table of the Dietary Reference Intakes (DRI) published by www.nap.edu.

TABLE A.15. DIETARY REFERENCE
INTAKES (DRI) OF MINERAL MANGANESE

Age	RDA/AI*	UL
	mg/d	mg/d
Infants		
0–6 mo	0.003*	ND
7–12 mo	0.6*	ND
Children		
1–3 y	1.2*	2
4–8 y	1.5*	3
Males		
9–13 y	1.9*	6
14–18 y	2.2*	9
19 y and up	2.3*	11
Females		
9–13 y	1.6*	6
14–18 y	1.6*	9
19 y and up	1.8*	11
Pregnancy		
under 18 y	2.0*	9
19–50 y	2.0*	11
Lactation		
under 18 y	2.6*	9
19–50 y	2.6*	11

RDA = Recommended Dietary Allowances
*AI = Adequate Intake
UL = Tolerable Upper Intake Value
ND = not determined
mg = milligram; d = day

The values are adapted and summarized from the table of the Dietary Reference Intakes (DRI) published by www.nap.edu.

TABLE A.16. DIETARY REFERENCE INTAKES (DRI) OF MINERAL CHROMIUM

Age	RDA/AI*	UL
	µg/d	µg/d
Infants		
0–6 mo	0.2*	ND
7–12 mo	5.5*	ND
Children		
1–3 y	11*	ND
4–8 y	15*	ND
Males		
9–13 y	25*	ND
14–50 y	35*	ND
51 y and up	30*	ND
Females		
9–13 y	21*	ND
14–18 y	24*	ND
19–50 y	25*	ND
Pregnancy		
under 18 y	29*	ND
19–50 y	30*	ND
Lactation		
under 18 y	44*	ND
19–50 y	45*	ND

RDA = Recommended Dietary Allowances
*AI = Adequate Intake
UL = Tolerable Upper Intake Value
ND = not determined
µg = microgram; d = day

The values are adapted and summarized from the table of the Dietary Reference Intakes (DRI) published by www.nap.edu.

TABLE A.17. DIETARY REFERENCE
INTAKES (DRI) OF MINERAL COPPER

Age	RDA/AI*	UL
	µg/d	µg/d
Infants		
0–6 mo	200*	ND
7–12 mo	220*	ND
Children		
1–3 y	340	1,000
4–8 y	440	3,000
Males		
9–13 y	700	5,000
14–18 y	890	8,000
19 y and up	900	10,000
Females		
9–13 y	700	5,000
14–18 y	890	8,000
19 y and up	900	10,000
Pregnancy		
under 18 y	1,000	8,000
19–50 y	1,000	10,000
Lactation		
under 18 y	1,300	8,000
19–50 y	1,300	10,000

RDA = Recommended Dietary Allowances
*AI = Adequate Intake
UL = Tolerable Upper Intake Value
ND = not determined
µg = microgram; d = day

The values are adapted and summarized from the table of the Dietary Reference Intakes (DRI) published by www.nap.edu.

TABLE A.18. DIETARY REFERENCE INTAKES (DRI) OF MINERAL IRON

Age	RDA/AI*	UL
	mg/d	mg/d
Infants		
0–6 mo	0.27*	40
7–12 mo	11	40
Children		
1–3 y	7	40
4–8 y	10	40
Males		
9–13 y	8	40
14–18 y	11	45
19 y and up	8	45
Females		
9–13 y	8	40
14–18 y	15	45
19–50 y	18	45
50 y and up	8	45
Pregnancy		
18–50 y	27	45
Lactation		
under 18 y	10	45
19–50 y	9	45

RDA = Recommended Dietary Allowances
*AI = Adequate Intake
UL = Tolerable Upper Intake Value
ND = not determined
mg = milligram; d = day

The values are adapted and summarized from the table of the Dietary Reference Intakes (DRI) published by www.nap.edu.

TABLE A.19. DIETARY REFERENCE
INTAKES (DRI) OF MINERAL SELENIUM

Age	RDA/AI*	UL
	µg/d	µg/d
Infants		
0–6 mo	15*	45
7–12 mo	20*	60
Children		
1–3 y	20	90
4–8 y	30	150
Males		
9–13 y	40	280
14 y and up	55	400
Females		
9–13 y	40	280
14 y and up	55	400
Pregnancy		
18–50 y	60	400
Lactation		
18–50 y	70	400

RDA = Recommended Dietary Allowances
*AI = Adequate Intake
UL = Tolerable Upper Intake Value
ND = not determined
µg = microgram; d = day

The values are adapted and summarized from the table of the Dietary Reference Intakes (DRI) published by www.nap.edu.

TABLE A.20. DIETARY REFERENCE INTAKES (DRI) OF MINERAL PHOSPHORUS

Age	RDA/AI*	UL
	mg/d	mg/d
Infants		
0–6 mo	100*	ND
7–12 mo	275*	ND
Children		
1–3 y	460	3,000
4–8 y	500	3,000
Males		
9–18 y	1,250	4,000
19–70 y	700	4,000
70 y and up	700	3,000
Females		
9–18 y	1,250	4,000
19–70 y	700	4,000
70 y and up	700	3,000
Pregnancy		
under 18 y	1,250	3,500
19–50 y	700	3,500
Lactation		
under 18 y	1,250	4,000
19–50 y	700	4,000

RDA = Recommended Dietary Allowances
*AI = Adequate Intake
UL = Tolerable Upper Intake Value
ND = not determined
mg = milligram; d = day

The values are adapted and summarized from the table of the Dietary Reference Intakes (DRI) published by www.nap.edu.

TABLE A.21. DIETARY REFERENCE INTAKES (DRI) OF MINERAL ZINC

Age	RDA/AI*	UL
	mg/d	mg/d
Infants		
0–6	2*	4
7–12 mo	3	5
Children		
1–3 y	3	7
4–8 y	5	12
Males		
9–13 y	8	23
14–18 y	11	34
19 y and up	11	40
Females		
9–13 y	8	23
14–18 y	9	34
19 y and up	8	40
Pregnancy		
under 18 y	12	34
19–50 y	11	40
Lactation		
under 18 y	13	34
19–50 y	12	40

RDA = Recommended Dietary Allowances
*AI = Adequate Intake
UL = Tolerable Upper Intake Value
ND = not determined
mg = milligram; d = day

The values are adapted and summarized from the table of the Dietary Reference Intakes (DRI) published by www.nap.edu.

TABLE A.22. CALORIE CONTENT
OF SELECTED FOODS

Food	Portion size	Calories
Apple	1	80
Banana	1	100
Beans, green cooked	½ cup	18
Bread, whole wheat	1 slice	56
Butter	1 tablespoon	100
Carrot	1 medium	34
Cheese	1 ounce	107–114
Corn on the cob	5½ inches	160
Egg	1 large	80
Ice cream	½ cup	135
Kidney beans, cooked	½ cup	110
Meat	3 ounces	200–250
Milk, skim	1 cup	85
Milk, whole	1 cup	150
Orange	1	65
Peach	1	38
Peanuts	1 ounce	172
Pear	1	100
Peas	½ cup	86
Potato chips	10 chips	115
Rice, cooked	½ cup	110
Shrimp	3 ounces	78
Tuna	3 ounces	78
Yogurt, low fat	1 cup	140

From K. N. Prasad and K. C. Prasad, *Fight Cancer with Vitamins and Supplements: A Guide to Prevention and Treatment*, Rochester, Vt.: Healing Arts Press, 2001.

TABLE A.23. FAT CONTENT
OF SELECTED FOODS

Food	Portion size	Grams/Portion
Avocado	⅛	4
Bacon, crisp	2 slices	6
Beef, roast	3 ounces	26
Biscuit	1	4
Bread, whole wheat	1 slice	1
Cheese, cheddar	1 ounce	9
Chicken, baked, with skin	3 ounces	11
Chicken, baked, without skin	3 ounces	6
Cornbread	1 piece	7
Egg, boiled	1	6
Ice cream	½ cup	7
Margarine	1 teaspoon	4
Mayonnaise	1 tablespoon	11
Milk, skim	1 cup	1
Milk, whole	1 cup	8
Oatmeal, cooked	½ cup	1
Peanut butter	1 tablespoon	7
Pork chop	3 ounces	19
Shrimp	3 ounces	0.9
Sour cream	1 tablespoon	3
Tuna	3 ounces	0.9
Vegetable oil	1 teaspoon	5
Yogurt, low fat	1 cup	4

From K. N. Prasad and K. C. Prasad, *Fight Cancer with Vitamins and Supplements: A Guide to Prevention and Treatment*, Rochester, Vt.: Healing Arts Press, 2001.

TABLE A.24. FIBER CONTENT
OF SELECTED FOODS

Food	Portion size	Grams/Portion
Apple, with skin	1	3
Bread, white	1 slice	0.8
Bread, whole wheat	1 slice	1.3
Broccoli	½ cup	3.2
Carrot, raw	1 medium	2.4
Cereal, all-bran	1 cup	25.6
Cereal, raisin bran	1 cup	6
Corn	½ cup	4.6
Muffin, bran	1	4.2
Pear, with skin	1	3.8
Raspberries	½ cup	4.6

From K. N. Prasad and K. C. Prasad, *Fight Cancer with Vitamins and Supplements: A Guide to Prevention and Treatment*, Rochester, Vt.: Healing Arts Press, 2001.

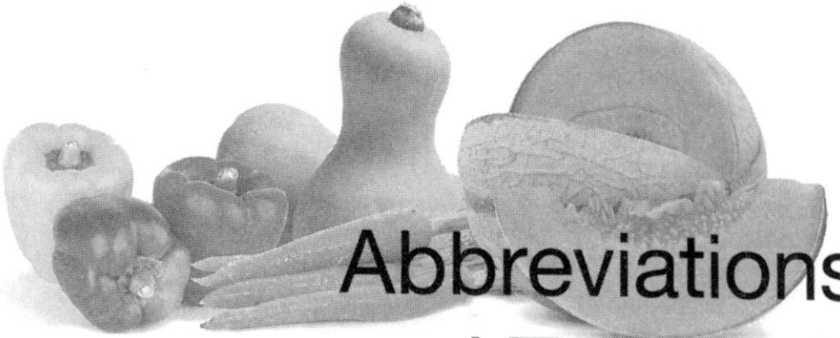

Abbreviations
and Terminologies

3-NP: 3-nitropropionic acid

3-NT: 3-nitrotyrosine

4-HNE: 4-hydroxynonenal

8-OHdG: 8-hydroxy-2-deoxyguanosine

Aß1-42: beta-amyloid fragments generated from APPP

APOE: apolipoprotein E

APP: amyloid precursor protein

ARE: antioxidant response element

BDNF: brain-derived neurotrophic factor

COX: cyclooxygenase

CRP: C-reactive protein

CSF: cerebrospinal fluid

DA: dopamine

EMF: electromagnetic field

EMP: electromagnetic pulse

GABA: gamma-aminobutyric acid

GDNF: glial cell-derived neurotrophic factor

GLT-1: glutamate transporter-1

GPX: glutathione peroxidase

H$_2$O$_2$: hydrogen peroxide

HO-1: heme oxygenase

IL-6: interleukin-6

MAO: monoamine oxidase

MCI: mild cognitive impairment

MDA: malondialdehyde

MPTP: 1-methyl-4-phenyl 1,2,3,6-tetrahydropyridine

MRI: magnetic resonance imaging

NAC: N-acetylcysteine

NAD: nicotinamide adenine dinucleotide

NADH: reduced form of NAD

NFkappaB: nuclear factor kappa-beta

NGF: nerve growth factor

NFT: neurofibrillary tangle

NMDA: N-methyl-D-aspartate

NO: nitric oxide

Nrf2: nuclear factor-erythroid 2-related factor 2

NSAID: nonsteroidal anti-inflammatory drug

PDH: pyruvate dehydrogenase

PET: positron emission tomography

P-tau: hyperphosphorylated tau protein

RBC: red blood cell

ROS: reactive oxygen species, also called free radicals

SelM: Selenoprotein M

SN: substantia nigra

SOD: superoxide dismutase

TBARS: thiobarbituric acid reactive substances

TNF-alpha: Tumor necrosis factor-alpha

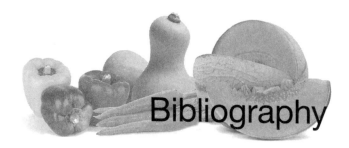

Bibliography

"1994–2004, The Development of DRIs: Lessoned Learned and New Challenges." 2008 Workshop. Washington, D.C.: National Academic Press.

Abate, A., G. Yang, P. A. Dennery, S. Oberle, and H. Schroder. 2000. Synergistic inhibition of cyclooxygenase-2 expression by vitamin E and aspirin. *Free Radic Biol Med* 29, no. 11: 135–42.

Abdul, H. M., R. Sultana, D. K. St. Clair, W. R. Markesbery, and D. A. Butterfield. 2008. Oxidative damage in brain from human mutant APP/PS-1 double knock-in mice as a function of age. *Free Radic Biol Med* 45, no. 10: 1420–5.

Aisen, P. S., K. L. Davis, J. D. Berg, et al. 2000. A randomized controlled trial of prednisone in Alzheimer's disease. Alzheimer's Disease Cooperative Study. *Neurology* 54, no. 3: 588–93.

Aisen, P. S., L. S. Schneider, M. Sano, et al. 2008. High-dose B vitamin supplementation and cognitive decline in Alzheimer disease: a randomized controlled trial. *JAMA* 300, no. 15: 1774–83.

Albanes, D., O. P. Heinonen, J. K. Huttunen, et al. 1995. Effects of alpha-tocopherol and beta-carotene supplements on cancer incidence in the Alpha-Tocopherol Beta-Carotene Cancer Prevention Study. *Am J Clin Nutr* 62, no. 6 Suppl: 1427S–30S.

Alberdi, E., A. Wyssenbach, M. Alberdi, et al. 2013. Ca(2+) -dependent endoplasmic reticulum stress correlates with astrogliosis in oligomeric amyloid beta-treated astrocytes and in a model of Alzheimer's disease. *Aging Cell* 12, no. 2: 292–302.

Alzheimer's Association 2013. www.alz.org/alzheimers_disease_facts_and_figures.asp#cost. Accessed January 16, 2015.

Ames, B. N., W. E. Durston, E. Yamasaki, and F. D. Lee. 1973. Carcinogens are mutagens: a simple test system combining liver homogenates for activation and bacteria for detection. *Proc Natl Acad Sci USA* 70, no. 8: 2281–85.

Ames, B. N., M. K. Shigenaga, and T. M. Hagen. 1993. Oxidants, antioxidants, and the degenerative diseases of aging. *Proc Natl Acad Sci USA* 90, no. 17: 7915–22.

Ames, B. N., M. Profet, and L. S. Gold. 1990. Dietary pesticides (99.99% all natural). *Proc Natl Acad Sci U S A* 87, no. 19: 7777–81.

Andersen, K., L. J. Launer, A. Ott, A. W. Hoes, M. M. Breteler, and A. Hofman. 1995. Do nonsteroidal anti-inflammatory drugs decrease the risk for Alzheimer's disease? The Rotterdam Study. *Neurology* 45, no. 8: 1441–45.

Anderson, J. J. B., R. Martin, and S. C. Garner. *Nutrition and Health: An Introduction.* Durham, N.C.: Carolina Academic Press, 2005.

Anekonda, T. S. 2006. Resveratrol—a boon for treating Alzheimer's disease? *Brain Res Rev* 52, no. 2: 316–26.

Arendash, G. W., T. Mori, M. Dorsey, R. Gonzalez, N. Tajiri, and C. Borlongan. 2012. Electromagnetic treatment to old Alzheimer's mice reverses beta-amyloid deposition, modifies cerebral blood flow, and provides selected cognitive benefit. *PLoS ONE* 7, no. 4: e35751.

Arendash, G. W., W. Schleif, K. Rezai-Zadeh, et al. 2006. Caffeine protects Alzheimer's mice against cognitive impairment and reduces brain beta-amyloid production. *Neuroscience* 142, no. 4: 941–52.

Asmus, K. D., and M. M. Bonifacic. 1994. "Free radical chemistry." In: *Exercise and Oxygen Toxicity.* Edited by C. K. Sen, L. Packer, and O. Hanninen. New York: Elsevier, 1994.

Augustin, S., G. Rimbach, K. Augustin, et al. 2009. Effect of a short- and long-term treatment with ginkgo biloba extract on amyloid precursor protein levels in a transgenic mouse model relevant to Alzheimer's disease. *Arch Biochem Biophys* 481, no. 2: 177–82.

Barger, S. W., M. E. Goodwin, M. M. Porter, and M. L. Beggs. 2007. Glutamate release from activated microglia requires the oxidative burst and lipid peroxidation. *J Neurochem* 101, no. 5: 1205–13.

Baum, L., and A. Ng. 2004. Curcumin interaction with copper and iron suggests one possible mechanism of action in Alzheimer's disease animal models. *J Alzheimers Dis* 6, no. 4: 367–77; discussion 443–9.

Baum, M. K., A. Campa, S. Lai, et al. 2013. Effect of micronutrient supplementation on disease progression in asymptomatic, antiretroviral-naive, HIV-infected adults in Botswana: a randomized clinical trial. *JAMA* 310, no. 20: 2154–63.

Behl, C., J. B. Davis, R. Lesley, and D. Schubert. 1994. Hydrogen peroxide mediates amyloid beta protein toxicity. *Cell* 77, no. 6: 817–27.

Behl, C., J. Davis, G. M. Cole, and D. Schubert. 1992. Vitamin E protects nerve cells from amyloid beta protein toxicity. *Biochem Biophys Res Commun* 186, no. 2: 944–50.

Bergstrom, P., H. C. Andersson, Y. Gao, et al. 2011. Repeated transient sulforaphane stimulation in astrocytes leads to prolonged Nrf2-mediated gene expression and protection from superoxide-induced damage. *Neuropharmacology* 60, no. 2–3: 343–53.

Bernardi, A., R. L. Frozza, A. Meneghetti, et al. 2012. Indomethacin-loaded lipid-core nanocapsules reduce the damage triggered by Abeta1-42 in Alzheimer's disease models. *Int J Nanomedicine* 7: 4927–42.

Bhat, N. R., and L. Thirumangalakudi. 2013. Increased Tau Phosphorylation and Impaired Brain Insulin/IGF Signaling in Mice Fed a High Fat/High Cholesterol Diet. *J Alzheimers Dis* 36, no. 4: 781–89.

Birkmayer, J. G. 1996. Coenzyme nicotinamide adenine dinucleotide: new therapeutic approach for improving dementia of the Alzheimer type. *Ann Clin Lab Sci* 26, no. 1: 1–9.

Birks, J., and L. Flicker. 2006. Donepezil for mild cognitive impairment. *Cochrane Database Syst Rev* 3: CD006104.

Bondy, S. C., and A. Truong. 1999. Potentiation of beta-folding of beta-amyloid peptide 25–35 by aluminum salts. *Neurosci Lett* 267, no. 1: 25–8.

Breitner, J. C., B. A. Gau, K. A. Welsh, et al. 1994. Inverse association of anti-inflammatory treatments and Alzheimer's disease: initial results of a co-twin control study. *Neurology* 44, no. 2: 227–32.

Brown, A. M., B. S. Kristal, M. S. Effron, et al. 2000. Zn2+ inhibits alpha-ketoglutarate-stimulated mitochondrial respiration and the isolated alpha-ketoglutarate dehydrogenase complex. *J Biol Chem* 275, no. 18: 13441–47.

Butterfield, D. A., K. Hensley, M. Harris, M. Mattson, and J. Carney. 1994. Beta-Amyloid peptide free radical fragments initiate synaptosomal lipoperoxidation in a sequence-specific fashion: implications to Alzheimer's disease. *Biochem Biophys Res Commun* 200, no. 2: 710–15.

Cadenas, E. P., and L. Packer. *Handbook of Antioxidants*. New York: Marcel Dekker, Inc., 1996.

Candelario-Jalil, E., R. S. Akundi, H. S. Bhatia, et al. 2006. Ascorbic acid enhances the inhibitory effect of aspirin on neuronal cyclooxygenase-2-mediated prostaglandin E2 production. *J Neuroimmunol* 174, no. 1–2: 39–51.

Carlson, D. A., A. R. Smith, S. J. Fischer, et al. 2007. The plasma pharmacokinetics of R-(+)-lipoic acid administered as sodium R-(+)-lipoate to healthy human subjects. *Altern Med Rev* 12, no. 4: 343–51.

Cervellati, C., E. Cremonini, C. Bosi, et al. 2013. Systemic oxidative stress in older patients with mild cognitive impairment or late onset Alzheimer's disease. *Curr Alzheimer Res* 10, no. 4: 365–72.

Chan, K., X. D. Han, and Y. W. Kan. 2001. An important function of Nrf2 in combating oxidative stress: detoxification of acetaminophen. *Proc Natl Acad Sci USA* 98, no. 8: 4611–16.

Chan, P. H., and R. A. Fishman. 1980. Transient formation of superoxide radicals in polyunsaturated fatty acid-induced brain swelling. *J Neurochem* 35, no. 4: 1004–7.

Charlton, K. E., T. L. Rabinowitz, L. N. Geffen, and M. A. Dhansay. 2004. Lowered plasma vitamin C, but not vitamin E, concentrations in dementia patients. *J Nutr Health Aging* 8, no. 2: 99–107.

Checler, F., C. A. da Costa, K. Ancolio, et al. 2000. Role of the proteasome in Alzheimer's disease. *Biochim Biophys Acta* 1502, no. 1: 133–8.

Chen, L., J. S. Richardson, J. E. Caldwell, and L. C. Ang. 1994. Regional brain activity of free radical defense enzymes in autopsy samples from patients with Alzheimer's disease and from nondemented controls. *Int J Neurosci* 75, no. 1–2: 83–90.

Chen, P., R. R. Wang, X. J. Ma, et al. 2013. Different Forms of Selenoprotein M Differentially Affect Abeta Aggregation and ROS Generation. *Int J Mol Sci* 14, no. 3: 4385–99.

Chen, R. S., C. C. Huang, and N. S. Chu. 1997. Coenzyme Q10 treatment in mitochondrial encephalomyopathies. Short-term double-blind, crossover study. *Eur Neurol* 37, no. 4: 212–8.

Chen, Y. B., J. Li, J. Y. Liu, et al. 2011. Effect of Electromagnetic Pulses (EMP) on associative learning in mice and a preliminary study of mechanism. *Int J Radiat Biol* 87, no. 12: 1147–54.

Chinta, S. J., and J. K. Andersen. 2005. Dopaminergic neurons. *Int J Biochem Cell Biol* 37, no. 5: 942–46.

Chiu, C. C., K. P. Su, T. C. Cheng, et al. 2008. The effects of omega-3 fatty acids monotherapy in Alzheimer's disease and mild cognitive impairment: a preliminary randomized double-blind placebo-controlled study. *Prog Neuropsychopharmacol Biol Psychiatry* 32, no. 6: 1538–44.

Choi, H. K., Y. R. Pokharel, S. C. Lim, et al. 2009. Inhibition of liver fibrosis by solubilized coenzyme Q10: Role of Nrf2 activation in inhibiting transforming growth factor-beta1 expression. *Toxicol Appl Pharmacol* 240, no. 3: 377–84.

Choi, S. H., S. Aid, L. Caracciolo, et al. 2013. Cyclooxygenase-1 inhibition reduces amyloid pathology and improves memory deficits in a mouse model of Alzheimer's disease. *J Neurochem* 124, no. 1: 59–68.

Clausen, A., X. Xu, X. Bi, and M. Baudry. 2012. Effects of the superoxide dismutase/catalase mimetic EUK-207 in a mouse model of Alzheimer's disease: protection against and interruption of progression of amyloid and tau pathology and cognitive decline. *J Alzheimers Dis* 30, no. 1: 183–208.

Coelho, F. G., T. M. Vital, A. M. Stein, et al. 2014. Acute aerobic exercise increases brain-derived neurotrophic factor levels in elderly with Alzheimer's disease. *J Alzheimers Dis* 39, no. 2: 401–8.

Cole, M. G., and J. F. Prchal. 1984. Low serum vitamin B_{12} in Alzheimer-type dementia. *Age Ageing* 13, no. 2: 101–5.

Combs, Jr., G. F. *The Vitamins: Fundamental Aspects in Nutrition & and Health*, 2nd Edition. San Diego: Academic Press, 1998.

Conrad, C. C., P. L. Marshall, J. M. Talent, et al. 2000. Oxidized proteins in Alzheimer's plasma. *Biochem Biophys Res Commun* 275, no. 2: 678–81.

Cote, S., P. H. Carmichael, R. Verreault, et al. 2012. Nonsteroidal anti-inflammatory drug use and the risk of cognitive impairment and Alzheimer's disease. *Alzheimers Dement* 8, no. 3: 219–26.

Cotran, R. S., V. Kumar, and T. Collins, ed. 1999. *Disease of immunity, Pathologic Basis of Disease.* New York: W. B. Saunders Company, 1999.

Coyle, J. T., and P. Puttfarcken. 1993. Oxidative stress, glutamate, and neurodegenerative disorders. *Science* 262, no. 5134: 689–95.

Cuajungco, M. P., and G. J. Lees. 1998. Nitric oxide generators produce accumulation of chelatable zinc in hippocampal neuronal perikarya. *Brain Res* 799, no. 1: 118–29.

Cui, B., L. Zhu, X. She, et al. 2012. Chronic noise exposure causes persistence of tau hyperphosphorylation and formation of NFT tau in the rat hippocampus and prefrontal cortex. *Exp Neurol* 238, no. 2: 122–9.

de la Monte, S. M., and J. R. Wands. 2006. Molecular indices of oxidative stress and mitochondrial dysfunction occur early and often progress with severity of Alzheimer's disease. *J Alzheimers Dis* 9, no. 2: 167–81.

DeKosky, S. T., J. D. Williamson, A. L. Fitzpatrick, et al. 2008. Ginkgo biloba for prevention of dementia: a randomized controlled trial. *JAMA* 300, no. 19: 2253–62.

Desrumaux, C., A. Pisoni, J. Meunier, et al. 2013. Increased amyloid-beta peptide-induced memory deficits in phospholipid transfer protein (PLTP) gene knockout mice. *Neuropsychopharmacology* 38, no. 5: 817–25.

Devaraj, S., R. Tang, B. Adams-Huet, et al. 2007. Effect of high-dose alpha-tocopherol supplementation on biomarkers of oxidative stress and inflammation and carotid atherosclerosis in patients with coronary artery disease. *Am J Clin Nutr* 86, no. 5: 1392–98.

Ding, Y., A. Qiao, Z. Wang, et al. 2008. Retinoic acid attenuates beta-amyloid deposition and rescues memory deficits in an Alzheimer's disease transgenic mouse model. *J Neurosci* 28, no. 45: 11622–34.

Du, X., H. Li, Z. Wang, et al. 2013. Selenoprotein P and selenoprotein M block Zn-mediated Abeta aggregation and toxicity. *Metallomics* 5, no. 7: 861–70.

Duits, F. H., M. I. Kester, P. G. Scheffer, et al. 2013. Increase in Cerebrospinal Fluid F2-Isoprostanes is Related to Cognitive Decline in APOE epsilon4 Carriers. *J Alzheimers Dis* 36, no. 3: 563–70.

Duthie, G. G., J. R. Arthur, and W. P. James. 1991. Effects of smoking and vitamin E on blood antioxidant status. *Am J Clin Nutr* 53, no. 4 Suppl: 1061S–1063S.

Eikelenboom, P., and F. C. Stam. 1982. Immunoglobulins and complement factors in senile plaques. An immunoperoxidase study. *Acta Neuropathol (Berl)* 57, no. 2–3: 239–42.

Engelhart, M. J., M. I. Geerlings, A. Ruitenberg, et al. 2002. Dietary intake of antioxidants and risk of Alzheimer disease. *JAMA* 287, no. 24: 3223–29.

Erickson, J. T., T. A. Brosenitsch, and D. M. Katz. 2001. Brain-derived neurotrophic factor and glial cell line-derived neurotrophic factor are required simultaneously for survival of dopaminergic primary sensory neurons in vivo. *J Neurosci* 21, no. 2: 581–89.

Evatt, M. L., M. R. Delong, N. Khazai, et al. 2008. Prevalence of vitamin d insufficiency in patients with Parkinson's disease and Alzheimer's disease. *Arch Neurol* 65, no. 10: 1348–52.

Farina, N., M. G. Isaac, A. R. Clark, et al. 2012. Vitamin E for Alzheimer's dementia and mild cognitive impairment. *Cochrane Database Syst Rev* 11: CD002854.

Farr, S. A., T. O. Price, W. A. Banks, et al. 2012. Effect of alpha-lipoic acid on memory, oxidation, and lifespan in SAMP8 mice. *J Alzheimers Dis* 32, no. 2: 447–55.

Farrer, L. A., L. A. Cupples, J. L. Haines, et al. 1997. Effects of age, sex, and ethnicity on the association between apolipoprotein E genotype and Alzheimer disease. A meta-analysis. APOE and Alzheimer Disease Meta Analysis Consortium. *JAMA* 278, no. 16: 1349–56.

Feng, Z., C. Qin, Y. Chang, and J. T. Zhang. 2006. Early melatonin supplementation alleviates oxidative stress in a transgenic mouse model of Alzheimer's disease. *Free Radic Biol Med* 40, no. 1: 101–9.

Fillenbaum, G. G., M. N. Kuchibhatla, J. T. Hanlon, et al. 2005. Dementia and Alzheimer's disease in community-dwelling elders taking vitamin C and/or vitamin E. *Ann Pharmacother* 39, no. 12: 2009–14.

Fleming, J. T., W. He, C. Hao, et al. 2013. The Purkinje neuron acts as a central regulator of spatially and functionally distinct cerebellar precursors. *Dev Cell* 27, no. 3: 278–92.

Fotuhi, M., P. Mohassel, and K. Yaffe. 2009. Fish consumption, long-chain omega-3 fatty acids and risk of cognitive decline or Alzheimer disease: a complex association. *Nat Clin Pract Neurol* 5, no. 3: 140–52.

Fotuhi, M., P. P. Zandi, K. M. Hayden, et al. 2008. Better cognitive performance in elderly taking antioxidant vitamins E and C supplements in combination with nonsteroidal anti-inflammatory drugs: the Cache County Study. *Alzheimers Dement* 4, no. 3: 223–27.

Frei, B. *Natural Antioxidants in Human Health and Disease.* New York: Academic Press, 1994.

Freund-Levi, Y., M. Eriksdotter-Jonhagen, T. Cederholm, et al. 2006. Omega-3 fatty acid treatment in 174 patients with mild to moderate Alzheimer disease: OmegAD study: a randomized double-blind trial. *Arch Neurol* 63, no. 10: 1402–8.

Frohman, E. M., T. C. Frohman, S. Gupta, et al. 1991. Expression of intercellular 1 (ICAM-1) in Alzheimer's disease. *J Neurol Sci* 106, no. 1: 105–11.

Fu, Y., S. Zheng, J. Lin, et al. 2008. Curcumin protects the rat liver from CCl4-caused injury and fibrogenesis by attenuating oxidative stress and suppressing inflammation. *Mol Pharmacol* 73, no. 2: 399–409.

Furio, A. M., L. I. Brusco, and D. P. Cardinali. 2007. Possible therapeutic value of melatonin in mild cognitive impairment: a retrospective study. *J Pineal Res* 43, no. 4: 404–9.

Gao, L., J. Wang, K. R. Sekhar, et al. 2007. Novel n-3 fatty acid oxidation products activate Nrf2 by destabilizing the association between Keap1 and Cullin3. *J Biol Chem* 282, no. 4: 2529–37.

Gaziano, J. M., H. D. Sesso, W. G. Christen, et al. 2012. Multivitamins in the prevention of cancer in men: the Physicians' Health Study II randomized controlled trial. *JAMA* 308, no. 18: 1871–80.

Gehrman, P. R., D. J. Connor, J. L. Martin, et al. 2009. Melatonin fails to improve sleep or agitation in double-blind randomized placebo-controlled trial of institutionalized patients with Alzheimer disease. *Am J Geriatr Psychiatry* 17, no. 2: 166–9.

Goedert, M., R. Jakes, R. A. Crowther, et al. 1993. The abnormal phosphorylation of tau protein at Ser-202 in Alzheimer disease recapitulates phosphorylation during development. *Proc Natl Acad Sci USA* 90, no. 11: 5066–70.

Graham, D. G. 1978. Oxidative pathways for catecholamines in the genesis of neuromelanin and cytotoxic quinones. *Mol Pharmacol* 14, no. 4: 633–43.

Gray, S. L., M. L. Anderson, P. K. Crane, et al. 2008. Antioxidant vitamin supplement use and risk of dementia or Alzheimer's disease in older adults. *J Am Geriatr Soc* 56, no. 2: 291–95.

Green, K. N., J. S. Steffan, H. Martinez-Coria, et al. 2008. Nicotinamide restores cognition in Alzheimer's disease transgenic mice via a mechanism involving sirtuin inhibition and selective reduction of Thr231-phosphotau. *J Neurosci* 28, no. 45: 11500–10.

Gregori, L., J. F. Hainfeld, M. N. Simon, and D. Goldgaber. 1997. Binding of amyloid beta protein to the 20 S proteasome. *J Biol Chem* 272, no. 1: 58–62.

Grundke-Iqbal, I., K. Iqbal, Y. C. Tung, et al. 1986. Abnormal phosphorylation of the microtubule-associated protein tau (tau) in Alzheimer cytoskeletal pathology. *Proc Natl Acad Sci USA* 83, no. 13: 4913–17.

Gu, X., J. Sun, S. Li, et al. 2013. Oxidative stress induces DNA demethylation and histone acetylation in SH-SY5Y cells: potential epigenetic mechanisms in gene transcription in Abeta production. *Neurobiol Aging* 34, no. 4: 1069–79.

Guo, C., P. Wang, M. L. Zhong, et al. 2013. Deferoxamine inhibits iron induced hippocampal tau phosphorylation in the Alzheimer transgenic mouse brain. *Neurochem Int* 62, no. 2: 165–72.

Guo, C., T. Wang, W. Zheng, et al. 2013. Intranasal deferoxamine reverses iron-induced memory deficits and inhibits amyloidogenic APP processing in a transgenic mouse model of Alzheimer's disease. *Neurobiol Aging* 34, no. 2: 562–75.

Haag, M. D., A. Hofman, P. J. Koudstaal, et al. 2009. Statins are associated with a reduced risk of Alzheimer disease regardless of lipophilicity. The Rotterdam Study. *J Neurol Neurosurg Psychiatry* 80, no. 1: 13–17.

Hager, K., M. Kenklies, J. McAfoose, et al. 2007. Alpha-lipoic acid as a new treatment option for Alzheimer's disease—a 48 months follow-up analysis. *J Neural Transm Suppl* 72: 189–93.

Hamaguchi, T., K. Ono, and M. Yamada. 2010. REVIEW: Curcumin and Alzheimer's disease. *CNS Neurosci Ther* 16, no. 5: 285–97.

Hamilton, R. L. 2000. Lewy bodies in Alzheimer's disease: a neuropathological review of 145 cases using alpha-synuclein immunohistochemistry. *Brain Pathol* 10, no. 3: 378–84.

Handattu, S. P., C. E. Monroe, G. Nayyar, et al. 2013. In vivo and in vitro effects of an apolipoprotein E mimetic peptide on amyloid-beta pathology. *J Alzheimers Dis* 36, no. 2: 335–47.

Harman, D. 1992. Free radical theory of aging. *Mutat Res* 275, no. 3–6: 257–66.

———. 1996. A hypothesis on the pathogenesis of Alzheimer's disease. *Ann NY Acad Sci* 786: 152–68.

Hartl, D., V. Schuldt, S. Forler, et al. 2012. Presymptomatic Alterations in Energy Metabolism and Oxidative Stress in the APP23 Mouse Model of Alzheimer Disease. *J Proteome Res* 11, no. 6: 3295–304.

Hayes, J. D., S. A. Chanas, C. J. Henderson, et al. 2000. The Nrf2 transcription factor contributes both to the basal expression of glutathione S-transferases in mouse liver and to their induction by the chemopreventive synthetic antioxidants, butylated hydroxyanisole and ethoxyquin. *Biochem Soc Trans* 28, no. 2: 33–41.

Hennekens, C. H., J. E. Buring, J. E. Manson, et al. 1996. Lack of effect of long-term supplementation with beta-carotene on the incidence of malignant neoplasm and cardiovascular disease. *N Eng J Med* 334: 1145–49.

Hine, C. M., and J. R. Mitchell. 2012. NRF2 and the Phase II Response in Acute Stress Resistance Induced by Dietary Restriction. *J Clin Exp Pathol* S4, no. 4.

Hiramatsu, M., R. D. Velasco, D. S. Wilson, and L. Packer. 1991. Ubiquinone protects against loss of tocopherol in rat liver microsomes and mitochondrial membranes. *Res Commun Chem Pathol Pharmacol* 72, no. 2: 231–41.

Hirohata, M., K. Ono, H. Naiki, and M. Yamada. 2005. Non-steroidal anti-inflammatory drugs have anti-amyloidogenic effects for Alzheimer's beta-amyloid fibrils in vitro. *Neuropharmacology* 49, no. 7: 1088–99.

Ho, Y. S., X. Yang, S. C. Yeung, et al. 2012. Cigarette smoking accelerated brain aging and induced pre-Alzheimer-like neuropathology in rats. *PLoS ONE* 7, no. 5: e36752.

Holland, E. C., and H. E. Varmus. 1998. Basic fibroblast growth factor induces cell migration and proliferation after glia-specific gene transfer in mice. *Proc Natl Acad Sci USA* 95, no. 3: 1218–23.

Holmquist, L., G. Stuchbury, K. Berbaum, et al. 2007. Lipoic acid as a novel treatment for Alzheimer's disease and related dementias. *Pharmacol Ther* 113, no. 1: 154–64.

Holtmeier, W., and D. Kabelitz. 2005. Gammadelta T cells link innate and adaptive immune responses. *Chem Immunol Allergy* 86: 151–83.

Houlgatte, R., M. Mallat, P. Brachet, and A. Prochiantz. 1989. Secretion of nerve growth factor in cultures of glial cells and neurons derived from different regions of the mouse brain. *J Neurosci Res* 24, no. 2: 143–52.

Ikeda, T., K. Yamamoto, K. Takahashi, et al. 1992. Treatment of Alzheimer-type dementia with intravenous mecobalamin. *Clin Ther* 14, no. 3: 426–37.

Iqbal, K., F. Liu, C. X. Gong, et al. 2009. Mechanisms of tau-induced neuro-degeneration. *Acta Neuropathol* 118, no. 1: 53–69.

Irwin, D. J., T. J. Cohen, M. Grossman, et al. 2012. Acetylated tau, a novel pathological signature in Alzheimer's disease and other tauopathies. *Brain* 135, Pt 3: 807–18.

Isaac, M. G., R. Quinn, and N. Tabet. 2008. Vitamin E for Alzheimer's disease and mild cognitive impairment. *Cochrane Database Syst Rev* 3: CD002854.

Itoh, K., T. Chiba, S. Takahashi, et al. 1997. An Nrf2/small Maf heterodimer mediates the induction of phase II detoxifying enzyme genes through antioxidant response elements. *Biochem Biophys Res Commun* 236, no. 2: 313–22.

Ji, L., R. Liu, X. D. Zhang, et al. 2010. N-acetylcysteine attenuates phosgene-induced acute lung injury via up-regulation of Nrf2 expression. *Inhal Toxicol* 22, no. 7: 535–42.

Jiang, D. P., J. Li, J. Zhang, et al. 2013. Electromagnetic pulse exposure induces overexpression of Beta amyloid protein in rats. *Arch Med Res* 44, no. 3: 178–84.

Jiang, T., X. L. Zhi, Y. H. Zhang, et al. 2012. Inhibitory effect of curcumin on the Al(III)-induced Abeta(4)(2) aggregation and neurotoxicity in vitro. *Biochim Biophys Acta* 1822, no. 8: 1207–15.

Jick, H., G. L. Zornberg, S. S. Jick, et al. 2000. Statins and the risk of dementia. *Lancet* 356, no. 9242: 1627–31.

Jimenez-Jimenez, F. J., F. de Bustos, J. A. Molina, et al. 1997. Cerebrospinal fluid levels of alpha-tocopherol (vitamin E) in Alzheimer's disease. *J Neural Transm* 104, no. 6–7: 703–10.

Jimenez-Jimenez, F. J., J. A. Molina, F. de Bustos, et al. 1999. Serum levels of beta-carotene, alpha-carotene and vitamin A in patients with Alzheimer's disease. *Eur J Neurol* 6, no. 4: 495–97.

Kandel, E. R., J. H. Schwartz, and T. M. Jessel. *Principles of Neural Science.* New York: McGraw-Hill, 2000.

Kanninen, K., T. M. Malm, H. K. Jyrkkanen, et al. 2008. Nuclear factor erythroid 2-related factor 2 protects against beta amyloid. *Mol Cell Neurosci* 39, no. 3: 302–13.

Kehrer, J. P., and C. V. Smith, ed. Free radicals in biology: sources, reactives, and roles in the etiology of human diseases. Edited by B. Frei, *Natural Antioxidants in Human Health and Disease.* New York: Academy Press, Inc., 1994.

Kehry, M. R., and P. D. Hodgkin. 1994. B-cell activation by helper T-cell membranes. *Crit Rev Immunol* 14, nos. 3–4: 221–38.

Khanna, A., M. Guo, M. Mehra, and W. Royal, 3rd. 2013. Inflammation and oxidative stress induced by cigarette smoke in Lewis rat brains. *J Neuroimmunol* 254, nos. 1–2: 69–75.

Kiyosawa, H., M. Suko, H. Okudaira, et al. 1990. Cigarette smoking induces formation of 8-hydroxydeoxyguanosine, one of the oxidative DNA damages in human peripheral leukocytes. *Free Radic Res Commun* 11, nos. 1–3: 23–7.

Kode, A., S. Rajendrasozhan, S. Caito, et al. 2008. Resveratrol induces glutathione synthesis by activation of Nrf2 and protects against cigarette smoke-mediated oxidative stress in human lung epithelial cells. *Am J Physiol Lung Cell Mol Physiol* 294, no. 3: L478–88.

Koh, J. Y., S. W. Suh, B. J. Gwag, et al. 1996. The role of zinc in selective neuronal death after transient global cerebral ischemia. *Science* 272, no. 5264: 1013–6.

Kosenko, E. A., G. Aliev, L. A. Tikhonova, et al. 2012. Antioxidant status and energy state of erythrocytes in Alzheimer dementia: probing for markers. *CNS Neurol Disord Drug Targets* 11, no. 7: 926–32.

Kroger, E., R. Verreault, P. H. Carmichael, et al. 2009. Omega-3 fatty acids and risk of dementia: the Canadian Study of Health and Aging. *Am J Clin Nutr* 90, no. 1: 184–92.

Kudo, T., K. Iqbal, R. Ravid, et al. 1994. Alzheimer disease: correlation of cerebro-spinal fluid and brain ubiquitin levels. *Brain Res* 639, no. 1: 1–7.

Kurata, T., K. Miyazaki, N. Morimoto, et al. 2013. Atorvastatin and pitavastatin reduce oxidative stress and improve IR/LDL-R signals in Alzheimer's disease. *Neurol Res* 35, no. 2: 193–205.

Lafon-Cazal, M., S. Pietri, M. Culcasi, and J. Bockaert. 1993. NMDA-dependent superoxide production and neurotoxicity. *Nature* 364, no. 6437: 535–7.

Lam, Y. A., C. M. Pickart, A. Alban, et al. 2000. Inhibition of the ubiquitin-proteasome system in Alzheimer's disease. *Proc Natl Acad Sci USA* 97, no. 18: 9902–6.

Langermans, J. A., W. L. Hazenbos, and R. van Furth. 1994. Antimicrobial functions of mononuclear phagocytes. *J Immunol Methods* 174, nos. 1–2:185–94.

Lee, H. S., K. K. Jung, J. Y. Cho, et al. 2007. Neuroprotective effect of curcumin is mainly mediated by blockade of microglial cell activation. *Pharmazie* 62, no. 12: 937–42.

Lee, T. M., M. L. Wong, B. W. Lau, et al. 2014. Aerobic exercise interacts with neurotrophic factors to predict cognitive functioning in adolescents. *Psychoneuroendocrinology* 39: 214–24.

Leppala, J. M., J. Virtamo, and R. Fogelholm. 2000. Controlled trail of alpha-tocopherol and beta-carotene supplements on stroke incidence and mortality in male smokers. *Arterioscler Thromb Vasc Biol* 20, no. 1: 230–35.

Leuner, K., K. Schulz, T. Schutt, et al. 2012. Peripheral mitochondrial dysfunction in Alzheimer's disease: focus on lymphocytes. *Mol Neurobiol* 46, no. 1: 194–204.

Li, X. H., C. Y. Li, J. M. Lu, et al. 2012. Allicin ameliorates cognitive deficits ageing-induced learning and memory deficits through enhancing of Nrf2 antioxidant signaling pathways. *Neurosci Lett* 514, no. 1: 46–50.

Liao, Y. F., B. J. Wang, H. T. Cheng, et al. 2004. Tumor necrosis factor-alpha, interleukin-1beta, and interferon-gamma stimulate gamma-secretase-mediated cleavage of amyloid precursor protein through a JNK-dependent MAPK pathway. *J Biol Chem* 279, no. 47: 49523–32.

Lim, G. P., F. Yang, T. Chu, et al. 2000. Ibuprofen suppresses plaque pathology and inflammation in a mouse model for Alzheimer's disease. *J Neurosci* 20, no. 15: 5709–14.

Lim, H. J., S. B. Shim, S. W. Jee, et al. 2013. Green tea catechin leads to global improvement among Alzheimer's disease-related phenotypes in NSE/hAPP-C105 Tg mice. *J Nutr Biochem* 24, no. 7: 1302–13.

Liraz, O., A. Boehm-Cagan, and D. M. Michaelson. 2013. ApoE4 induces Abeta42, tau, and neuronal pathology in the hippocampus of young targeted replacement apoE4 mice. *Mol Neurodegener* 8:16.

Litman, G. W., J. P. Cannon, and L. J. Dishaw. 2005. Reconstructing immune phylogeny: new perspectives. *Nat Rev Immunol* 5, no. 11: 866–79.

Liu, B., A. Moloney, S. Meehan, et al. 2011. Iron promotes the toxicity of amyloid beta peptide by impeding its ordered aggregation. *J Biol Chem* 286, no. 6: 4248–56.

Liu, D., M. Pitta, H. Jiang, et al. 2013. Nicotinamide forestalls pathology and cognitive decline in Alzheimer mice: evidence for improved neuronal bioenergetics and autophagy procession. *Neurobiol Aging* 34, no. 6: 1564–80.

Liu, D., M. Pitta, and M. P. Mattson. 2008. Preventing NAD(+) depletion protects neurons against excitotoxicity: bioenergetic effects of mild mitochondrial uncoupling and caloric restriction. *Ann NY Acad Sci* 1147: 275–82.

Lopez Salon, M., L. Morelli, E. M. Castano, et al. 2000. Defective ubiquitination of cerebral proteins in Alzheimer's disease. *J Neurosci Res* 62, no. 2: 302–10.

Lopez, O. L., J. A. Mackell, Y. Sun, et al. 2008. Effectiveness and safety of donepezil in Hispanic patients with Alzheimer's disease: a 12-week open-label study. *J Natl Med Assoc* 100, no. 11: 1350–58.

Lopez-Pousa, S., A. Turon-Estrada, J. Garre-Olmo, et al. 2005. Differential efficacy of treatment with acetylcholinesterase inhibitors in patients with mild and moderate Alzheimer's disease over a 6-month period. *Dement Geriatr Cogn Disord* 19, no. 4: 189–95.

Lorenzo, A., and B. A. Yankner. 1994. Beta-amyloid neurotoxicity requires fibril formation and is inhibited by congo red. *Proc Natl Acad Sci USA* 91, no. 25: 12243–47.

Lucas, H. R., and J. M. Rifkind. 2013. Considering the vascular hypothesis of Alzheimer's disease: effect of copper associated amyloid on red blood cells. *Adv Exp Med Biol* 765: 131–38.

Lucca, U., M. Tettamanti, G. Forloni, and A. Spagnoli. 1994. Nonsteroidal antiinflammatory drug use in Alzheimer's disease. *Biol Psychiatry* 36, no. 12: 854–56.

Luchsinger, J. A., M. X. Tang, M. Siddiqui, et al. 2004. Alcohol intake and risk of dementia. *J Am Geriatr Soc* 52, no. 4: 540–6.

Ma, W. W., C. C. Hou, X. Zhou, et al. 2013. Genistein alleviates the mitochondria-targeted DNA damage induced by beta-amyloid peptides 25–35 in C6 glioma cells. *Neurochem Res* 38, no. 7: 1315–23.

Mackenzie, I. R., and D. G. Munoz. 1998. Nonsteroidal anti-inflammatory drug use and Alzheimer-type pathology in aging. *Neurology* 50, no. 4: 986–90.

Maczurek, A., K. Hager, M. Kenklies, et al. 2008. Lipoic acid as an anti-inflammatory and neuroprotective treatment for Alzheimer's disease. *Adv Drug Deliv Rev* 60, nos. 13–14: 1463–70.

Malouf, R., and J. Grimley Evans. 2008. Folic acid with or without vitamin B_{12} for the prevention and treatment of healthy elderly and demented people. *Cochrane Database Syst Rev* 4: CD004514.

Marambaud, P., H. Zhao, and P. Davies. 2005. Resveratrol promotes clearance of Alzheimer's disease amyloid-beta peptides. *J Biol Chem* 280, no. 45: 37377–82.

Martin, B. K., C. Szekely, J. Brandt, et al. 2008. Cognitive function over time in the Alzheimer's Disease Anti-inflammatory Prevention Trial (ADAPT): results of a randomized, controlled trial of naproxen and celecoxib. *Arch Neurol* 65, no. 7: 896–905.

Martin, P., and S. J. Leibovich. 2005. Inflammatory cells during wound repair: the good, the bad and the ugly. *Trends Cell Biol* 15, no. 11: 599–607.

Marx, J. 1998. New gene tied to common form of Alzheimer's. *Science* 281, no. 5376: 507, 509.

Matzinger, P. 2002. The danger model: a renewed sense of self. *Science* 296, no. 5566: 301–5.

McConnell, L. M., B. A. Koenig, H. T. Greely, and T. A. Raffin. 1998.

Genetic testing and Alzheimer disease: has the time come? Alzheimer Disease Working Group of the Stanford Program in Genomics, Ethics & Society. *Nat Med* 4, no. 7: 757–59.

McDonald, S. R., R. S. Sohal, and M. J. Forster. 2005. Concurrent administration of coenzyme Q10 and alpha-tocopherol improves learning in aged mice. *Free Radic Biol Med* 38, no. 6: 729–36.

McGeer, E. G., and P. L. McGeer. 1998. The importance of inflammatory mechanisms in Alzheimer's disease. *Exp Gerontol* 33, no. 5: 371–78.

McGeer, P. L. 2000. Cyclo-oxygenase-2 inhibitors: rationale and therapeutic potential for Alzheimer's disease. *Drugs Aging* 17, no. 1: 1–11.

McKee, A. C., I. Carreras, L. Hossain, et al. 2008. Ibuprofen reduces Abeta, hyperphosphorylated tau and memory deficits in Alzheimer mice. *Brain Res* 1207: 225–36.

Medzhitov, R. 2007. Recognition of microorganisms and activation of the immune response. *Nature* 449, no. 7164: 819–26.

Melov, S., P. A. Adlard, K. Morten, et al. 2007. Mitochondrial oxidative stress causes hyperphosphorylation of tau. *PLoS ONE* 2, no. 6: e536.

Misonou, H., M. Morishima-Kawashima, and Y. Ihara. 2000. Oxidative stress induces intracellular accumulation of amyloid beta-protein (Abeta) in human neuroblastoma cells. *Biochemistry* 39, no. 23: 6951–59.

Mohmmad Abdul, H., R. Sultana, J. N. Keller, et al. 2006. Mutations in amyloid precursor protein and presenilin-1 genes increase the basal oxidative stress in murine neuronal cells and lead to increased sensitivity to oxidative stress mediated by amyloid beta-peptide (1–42), HO and kainic acid: implications for Alzheimer's disease. *J Neurochem* 96, no. 5: 1322–35.

Moreira, P. I., P. L. Harris, X. Zhu, et al. 2007. Lipoic acid and N-acetyl cysteine decrease mitochondrial-related oxidative stress in Alzheimer disease patient fibroblasts. *J Alzheimers Dis* 12, no. 2: 195–206.

Moreira, P. I., M. S. Santos, C. Sena, et al. 2005. CoQ10 therapy attenuates amyloid beta-peptide toxicity in brain mitochondria isolated from aged diabetic rats. *Exp Neurol* 196, no. 1: 112–19.

Mota, S. I., I. L. Ferreira, C. Pereira, et al. 2012. Amyloid-beta peptide 1-42 causes microtubule deregulation through N-methyl-D-aspartate receptors in mature hippocampal cultures. *Curr Alzheimer Res* 9, no. 7: 844–56.

Mucha, L., S. Shaohung, B. Cuffel, et al. 2008. Comparison of cholinesterase inhibitor utilization patterns and associated health care costs in Alzheimer's disease. *J Manag Care Pharm* 14, no. 5: 451–61.

Murakami, K., N. Murata, Y. Noda, et al. 2012. Stimulation of the amyloidogenic pathway by cytoplasmic superoxide radicals in an Alzheimer's disease mouse model. *Biosci Biotechnol Biochem* 76, no. 6: 1098–103.

Mutisya, E. M., A. C. Bowling, and M. F. Beal. 1994. Cortical cytochrome oxidase activity is reduced in Alzheimer's disease. *J Neurochem* 63, no. 6: 2179–84.

Nahreini, P., C. Andreatta, and K. N. Prasad. 2001. Proteasome activity is critical for the cAMP-induced differentiation of neuroblastoma cells. *Cell Mol Neurobiol* 21, no. 5: 509–21.

Naslund, J., V. Haroutunian, R. Mohs, et al. 2000. Correlation between elevated levels of amyloid beta-peptide in the brain and cognitive decline. *JAMA* 283, no. 12: 1571–77.

Niki, E. 1997. Mechanisms and dynamics of antioxidant action of ubiquinol. *Mol. Aspects Med* 18 (suppl): S63–S70.

Niture, S. K., J. W. Kaspar, J. Shen, and A. K. Jaiswal. 2010. Nrf2 signaling and cell survival. *Toxicol Appl Pharmacol* 244, no. 1: 37–42.

Olcese, J. M., C. Cao, T. Mori, et al. 2009. Protection against cognitive deficits and markers of neurodegeneration by long-term oral administration of melatonin in a transgenic model of Alzheimer disease. *J Pineal Res* 47, no. 1: 82–96.

Ono, K., K. Hasegawa, H. Naiki, and M. Yamada. 2005. Preformed beta-amyloid fibrils are destabilized by coenzyme Q10 in vitro. *Biochem Biophys Res Commun* 330, no. 1: 111–16.

Ono, K., Y. Yoshiike, A. Takashima, et al. 2004. Vitamin A exhibits potent antiamyloidogenic and fibril-destabilizing effects in vitro. *Exp Neurol* 189, no. 2: 380–92.

Packer, L., M. Hiramatsu, and T. Yoshikawa. *Antioxidants Food Supplements in Human Health.* New York: Academic Press, 1999.

Parent, A., and M. B. Carpenter. *Carpenter's Human Anatomy.* Philadelphia: Williams & Wilkins, 1995.

Peairs, A. T., and J. W. Rankin. 2008. Inflammatory Response to a High-fat, Low-carbohydrate Weight Loss Diet: Effect of Antioxidants. *Obesity (Silver Spring)* 16, no. 7: 1573–78.

Peng, Q. L., A. R. Buzzard, and B. H. Lau. 2002. Pycnogenol protects neurons from amyloid-beta peptide-induced apoptosis. *Brain Res Mol Brain Res* 104, no. 1: 55–65.

Piaceri, I., V. Rinnoci, S. Bagnoli, et al. 2012. Mitochondria and Alzheimer's disease. *J Neurol Sci* 322, nos. 1–2: 31–34.

Placanica, L., L. Tarassishin, G. Yang, et al. 2009. Pen2 and presenilin-1 modulate the dynamic equilibrium of presenilin-1 and presenilin-2 gamma-secretase complexes. *J Biol Chem* 284, no. 5: 2967–77.

Prasad, K. N. *Micronutrients in Health and Disease.* Boca Raton, Fla.: CRC Press, 2011.

Prasad, K. N., A. R. Hovland, F. G. La Rosa, and P. G. Hovland. 1998. Prostaglandins as putative neurotoxins in Alzheimer's disease. *Proc Soc Exp Biol Med* 219, no. 2: 120–25.

Prasad, K. N., W. C. Cole, and K. C. Prasad. 2002. Risk factors for Alzheimer's disease: role of multiple antioxidants, non-steroidal anti-inflammatory and cholinergic agents alone or in combination in prevention and treatment. *J Am Coll Nutr* 21, no. 6: 506–22.

Prasad, K. N., and S. C. Bondy. 2014. Inhibiton of early upstream events in prodromal Alzheimer's disease by use of targeted Antioxidants. *Curr Aging Sci* 7: 1–14.

Prior, M., R. Dargusch, J. L. Ehren, et al. 2013. The neurotrophic compound J147 reverses cognitive impairment in aged Alzheimer's disease mice. *Alzheimers Res Ther* 5, no. 3: 25.

Pryor, W. A., ed. Oxidants and antioxidants. Edited by B. Frei, *Natural Antioxidants in Human Health and Disease.* New York: Academy Press, Inc., 1994.

Quinn, J. F., J. R. Bussiere, R. S. Hammond, et al. 2007. Chronic dietary alpha-lipoic acid reduces deficits in hippocampal memory of aged Tg2576 mice. *Neurobiol Aging* 28, no. 2: 213–25.

Rahman, S., K. Bhatia, A. Q. Khan, et al. 2008. Topically applied vitamin E prevents massive cutaneous inflammatory and oxidative stress responses induced by double application of 12-O-tetradecanoylphorbol-13-acetate (TPA) in mice. *Chem Biol Interact* 172, no. 3: 195–205.

Rainer, M., E. Kraxberger, M. Haushofer, et al. 2000. No evidence for cognitive improvement from oral nicotinamide adenine dinucleotide (NADH) in dementia. *J Neural Transm* 107, no. 12: 1475–81.

Ramirez, G., S. Rey, and R. von Bernhardi. 2008. Proinflammatory stimuli are needed for induction of microglial cell-mediated AbetaPP_{244-C} and Abeta-neurotoxicity in hippocampal cultures. *J Alzheimers Dis* 15, no. 1: 45–59.

Ramsey, C. P., C. A. Glass, M. B. Montgomery, et al. 2007. Expression of Nrf2 in neurodegenerative diseases. *J Neuropathol Exp Neurol* 66, no. 1: 75–85.

Refolo, L. M., B. Malester, J. LaFrancois, et al. 2000. Hypercholesterolemia accelerates the Alzheimer's amyloid pathology in a transgenic mouse model. *Neurobiol Dis* 7, no. 4: 321–31.

Rezai-Zadeh, K., G. W. Arendash, H. Hou, et al. 2008. Green tea epigallocatechin-3-gallate (EGCG) reduces beta-amyloid mediated cognitive impairment and modulates tau pathology in Alzheimer transgenic mice. *Brain Res* 1214: 177–87.

Reznick, A. Z., C. E. Cross, M. L. Hu, et al. 1992. Modification of plasma proteins by cigarette smoke as measured by protein carbonyl formation. *Biochem J* 286, Pt 2: 607–11.

Rich, J. B., D. X. Rasmusson, M. F. Folstein, et al. 1995. Nonsteroidal anti-inflammatory drugs in Alzheimer's disease. *Neurology* 45, no. 1: 51–55.

Rinaldi, P., M. C. Polidori, A. Metastasio, et al. 2003. Plasma antioxidants are similarly depleted in mild cognitive impairment and in Alzheimer's disease. *Neurobiol Aging* 24, no. 7: 915–19.

Ringman, J. M., A. T. Fithian, K. Gylys, et al. 2012. Plasma methionine sulfoxide in persons with familial Alzheimer's disease mutations. *Dement Geriatr Cogn Disord* 33, no. 4: 219–25.

Rogers, J., L. C. Kirby, S. R. Hempelman, et al. 1993. Clinical trial of indomethacin in Alzheimer's disease. *Neurology* 43, no. 8: 1609–11.

Rogers, J., L-F. Lue, L. Brachova, et al. 1995. Inflammation as a response and a cause of Alzheimer's pathophysiology. *Dementia* 9: 133–38.

Rondeau, V., H. Jacqmin-Gadda, D. Commenges, et al. 2009. Aluminum and silica in drinking water and the risk of Alzheimer's disease or cognitive decline: findings from 15-year follow-up of the PAQUID cohort. *Am J Epidemiol* 169, no. 4: 489–96.

Rozemuller, J. M., P. Eikelenboom, S. T. Pals, and F. C. Stam. 1989. Microglial cells around amyloid plaques in Alzheimer's disease express leucocyte adhesion molecules of the LFA-1 family. *Neurosci Lett* 101, no. 3: 288–92.

Rus, H., C. Cudrici, and F. Niculescu. 2005. The role of the complement system in innate immunity. *Immunol Res* 33, no. 2: 103–12.

Ryter, A. 1985. Relationship between ultrastructure and specific functions of macrophages. *Comp Immunol Microbiol Infect Dis* 8, no. 2: 119–33.

Sainati, S., D. Ingram, and S. Talwalker. 2000. Results of a double-blind, placebo-controlled study of Celecoxib in the treatment of progression of Alzheimer's disease. Paper read at Sixth International Stockholm-Spingfield Symposium of Advances in Alzheimer's Therapy, at Stockholm.

Sandhu, J. K., S. Pandey, M. Ribecco-Lutkiewicz, et al. 2003. Molecular mechanisms of glutamate neurotoxicity in mixed cultures of NT2-derived neurons and astrocytes: protective effects of coenzyme Q10. *J Neurosci Res* 72, no. 6: 691–703.

Sano, M., C. Ernesto, R. G. Thomas, et al. 1997. A controlled trial of selegiline, alpha-tocopherol, or both as treatment for Alzheimer's disease. The Alzheimer's Disease Cooperative Study. *N Engl J Med* 336, no. 17: 1216–22.

Savaskan, E., G. Olivieri, F. Meier, et al. 2003. Red wine ingredient resveratrol protects from beta-amyloid neurotoxicity. *Gerontology* 49, no. 6: 380–83.

Saw, C. L., A. Y. Yang, Y. Guo, and A. N. Kong. 2013. Astaxanthin and omega-3 fatty acids individually and in combination protect against oxidative stress via the Nrf2-ARE pathway. *Food Chem Toxicol* 62: 869–75.

Scharf, S., A. Mander, A. Ugoni, et al. 1999. A double-blind, placebo-controlled trial of diclofenac/misoprostol in Alzheimer's disease. *Neurology* 53, no. 1: 197–201.

Schectman, G., J. C. Byrd, and R. Hoffmann. 1991. Ascorbic acid requirements for smokers: analysis of a population survey. *Am J Clin Nutr* 53, no. 6: 1466–70.

Schubert, D., C. Behl, R. Lesley, et al. 1995. Amyloid peptides are toxic via a common oxidative mechanism. *Proc Natl Acad Sci USA* 92, no. 6: 1989–93.

Schubert, D., H. Kimura, and P. Maher. 1992. Growth factors and vitamin E modify neuronal glutamate toxicity. *Proc Natl Acad Sci USA* 89, no. 17: 8264–67.

Selkoe, D. J. 1994. Cell biology of the amyloid beta-protein precursor and the mechanism of Alzheimer's disease. *Annu Rev Cell Biol* 10: 373–403.

Sen, C. K., L. Packer, and P. A. Baeuerle. *Antioxidants and Redox Regulation of Genes.* New York: Academic Press, 1999.

Shalit, F., B. Sredni, L. Stern, et al. 1994. Elevated interleukin-6 secretion levels by mononuclear cells of Alzheimer's patients. *Neurosci Lett* 174, no. 2: 130–2.

Sharif, S. F., R. J. Hariri, V. A. Chang, et al. 1993. Human astrocyte production of tumour necrosis factor-alpha, interleukin-1 beta, and interleukin-6 following exposure to lipopolysaccharide endotoxin. *Neurol Res* 15, no. 2: 109–12.

Sherrington, R., E. I. Rogaev, Y. Liang, et al. 1995. Cloning of a gene bearing missense mutations in early-onset familial Alzheimer's disease. *Nature* 375, no. 6534: 754–60.

Shils, M. E., M. Shike, A. C. Ross, et al. *Modern Nutrition in Health and Disease*, 10th Edition. Philadelphia: Lippincott Williams & Wilkins, 2005.

Shoffner, J. M., M. D. Brown, A. Torroni, et al. 1993. Mitochondrial DNA variants observed in Alzheimer's disease and Parkinson's disease patients. *Genomics* 17, no. 1: 171–84.

Shoulson, I. 1998. DATATOP: a decade of neuroprotective inquiry. Parkinson Study Group. Deprenyl And Tocopherol Antioxidative Therapy Of Parkinsonism. *Ann Neurol* 44, no. 3, Suppl 1: S160–66.

Siedlak, S. L., G. Casadesus, K. M. Webber, et al. 2009. Chronic antioxidant therapy reduces oxidative stress in a mouse model of Alzheimer's disease. *Free Radic Res* 43 (2): 156–64.

Smith, M. A., L. M. Sayre, V. M. Monnier, and G. Perry. 1995. Radical Ageing in Alzheimer's disease. *Trends Neurosci* 18, no. 4: 172–76.

Sochocka, M., E. S. Koutsouraki, K. Gasiorowski, and J. Leszek. 2013. Vascular oxidative stress and mitochondrial failure in the pathobiology of Alzheimer's disease: New approach to therapy. *CNS Neurol Disord Drug Targets* 12, no. 6: 870–81.

Sompol, P., W. Ittarat, J. Tangpong, et al. 2008. A neuronal model of Alzheimer's disease: an insight into the mechanisms of oxidative stress-mediated mitochondrial injury. *Neuroscience* 153, no. 1: 120–30.

Souza, L. C., C. B. Filho, A. T. Goes, et al. 2013. Neuroprotective Effect of Physical Exercise in a Mouse Model of Alzheimer's Disease Induced by beta-Amyloid(1-40) Peptide. *Neurotox Res* 24, no. 2: 148–63.

Sparks, D. L., T. A. Martin, D. R. Gross, and J. C. Hunsaker, 3rd. 2000. Link between heart disease, cholesterol, and Alzheimer's disease: a review. *Microsc Res Tech* 50, no. 4: 287–90.

Sproul, T. W., P. C. Cheng, M. L. Dykstra, and S. K. Pierce. 2000. A role for MHC class II antigen processing in B cell development. *Int Rev Immunol* 19, nos. 2–3: 139–55.

Steele, M. L., S. Fuller, M. Patel, et al. 2013. Effect of Nrf2 activators on release of glutathione, cysteinylglycine and homocysteine by human U373 astroglial cells. *Redox Biol* 1, no. 1: 441–45.

Suchy, J., A. Chan, and T. B. Shea. 2009. Dietary supplementation with a combination of alpha-lipoic acid, acetyl-L-carnitine, glycerophospho-coline, docosahexaenoic acid, and phosphatidylserine reduces oxidative damage to murine brain and improves cognitive performance. *Nutr Res* 29, no. 1: 70–74.

Suh, J. H., S. V. Shenvi, B. M. Dixon, et al. 2004. Decline in transcriptional activity of Nrf2 causes age-related loss of glutathione synthesis, which is reversible with lipoic acid. *Proc Natl Acad Sci USA* 101, no. 10: 3381–86.

Sultana, R., and D. A. Butterfield. 2009. Oxidatively modified, mitochondria-relevant brain proteins in subjects with Alzheimer disease and mild cognitive impairment. *J Bioenerg Biomembr* 41, no. 5: 441–46.

Sultana, R., M. Perluigi, and D. A. Butterfield. 2006. Protein oxidation and lipid peroxidation in brain of subjects with Alzheimer's disease: insights into mechanism of neurodegeneration from redox proteomics. *Antioxid Redox Signal* 8, nos. 11–12: 2021–37.

Sung, S., Y. Yao, K. Uryu, et al. 2004. Early vitamin E supplementation in young but not aged mice reduces Abeta levels and amyloid deposition in a transgenic model of Alzheimer's disease. *FASEB J* 18, no. 2: 323–25.

Sutton, E. T., T. Thomas, M. W. Bryant, et al. 1999. Amyloid-beta peptide induced inflammatory reaction is mediated by the cytokines tumor necrosis factor and interleukin-1. *J Submicrosc Cytol Pathol* 31, no. 3: 313–23.

Suzuki, Y. J., B. B. Aggarwal, and L. Packer. 1992. Alpha-lipoic acid is a potent inhibitor of NF-kappa B activation in human T cells. *Biochem Biophys Res Commun* 189, no. 3: 1709–15.

Tabaton, M., and E. Tamagno. 2007. The molecular link between beta- and gamma-secretase activity on the amyloid beta precursor protein. *Cell Mol Life Sci* 64, no. 17: 2211–18.

Tai, H. C., A. Serrano-Pozo, T. Hashimoto, et al. 2012. The synaptic accumulation of hyperphosphorylated tau oligomers in Alzheimer disease is associated with dysfunction of the ubiquitin-proteasome system. *Am J Pathol* 181, no. 4: 1426–35.

Tamminga, C., T. Hashimoto, D. W. Volk, and D. A. Lewis. 2004. GABA neurons in the human prefrontal cortex. *Am J Psychiatry* 161, no. 10: 1764.

Taylor, M., S. Moore, S. Mourtas, et al. 2011. Effect of curcumin-associated and lipid ligand-functionalized nanoliposomes on aggregation of the Alzheimer's Abeta peptide. *Nanomedicine* 7, no. 5: 541–50.

Tesco, G., S. Latorraca, P. Piersanti, et al. 1992. Alzheimer skin fibroblasts show increased susceptibility to free radicals. *Mech Ageing Dev* 66, no. 2: 117–20.

Thirumangalakudi, L., A. Prakasam, R. Zhang, et al. 2008. High cholesterol-induced neuroinflammation and amyloid precursor protein processing correlate with loss of working memory in mice. *J Neurochem* 106, no. 1: 475–85.

Thompson, R. F. *The Barin: An Introduction to Neuroscience.* Worth Publisher, 2000.

Toro, R., M. Perron, B. Pike, et al. 2008. Brain size and folding of the human cerebral cortex. *Cereb Cortex* 18, no. 10: 2352–57.

Torres, L. L., N. B. Quaglio, G. T. de Souza, et al. 2011. Peripheral oxidative stress biomarkers in mild cognitive impairment and Alzheimer's disease. *J Alzheimers Dis* 26, no. 1: 59–68.

Trujillo, J., Y. I. Chirino, E. Molina-Jijon, et al. 2013. Renoprotective effect of the antioxidant curcumin: Recent findings. *Redox Biol* 1, no. 1: 448–56.

Tornwall, M. E., J. Virtamo, P. A. Korhonen, et al. 2004a. Effect of alpha-tocopherol and beta-carotene supplementation on coronary heart disease during the 6-year post-trail follow-up in the ATBC study. *Eur heart J* 25, no. 13: 1171–78.

Tornwall, M. E., J. Virtamo, P. A. Korhonen, et al. 2004b. Postintervention effect of alpha-tocopherol and beta-carotene on different strokes: a 6-year follow-up of the Alpha Tocopherol, Beta carotene Cancer Prevention Study, *Stroke* 35, no. 8: 1908–13.

U.S. Census Bureau, U.S. Department of Commerce, 2010. www.census.gov/prod/2010pubs/p25-1138.pdf. Accessed January 16, 2015.

Vaillancourt, F., H. Fahmi, Q. Shi, et al. 2008. 4-Hydroxynonenal induces apoptosis in human osteoarthritic chondrocytes: the protective role of glutathione-S-transferase. *Arthritis Res Ther* 10, no. 5: R107.

van Dyck, C. H., J. M. Lyness, R. M. Rohrbaugh, and A. P. Siegal. 2009. Cognitive and psychiatric effects of vitamin B_{12} replacement in dementia with low serum B_{12} levels: a nursing home study. *Int Psychogeriatr* 21, no. 1: 138–47.

Varadarajan, S., S. Yatin, J. Kanski, et al. 1999. Methionine residue 35 is important in amyloid beta-peptide-associated free radical oxidative stress. *Brain Res Bull* 50, no. 2: 133–41.

Verbeek, M. M., I. Otte-Holler, J. R. Westphal, et al. 1994. Accumulation of intercellular adhesion molecule-1 in senile plaques in brain tissue of patients with Alzheimer's disease. *Am J Pathol* 144, no. 1: 104–16.

Vingtdeux, V., U. Dreses-Werringloer, H. Zhao, et al. 2008. Therapeutic potential of resveratrol in Alzheimer's disease. *BMC Neurosci* 9, Suppl 2: S6.

Wallace, D. C. 1992. Mitochondrial genetics: a paradigm for aging and degenerative diseases? *Science* 256, no. 5057: 628–32.

Wang, J., L. Ho, Z. Zhao, et al. 2006. Moderate consumption of Cabernet Sauvignon attenuates Abeta neuropathology in a mouse model of Alzheimer's disease. *FASEB J* 20, no. 13: 2313–20.

Webster, S., S. O'Barr, and J. Rogers. 1994. Enhanced aggregation and beta structure of amyloid beta peptide after coincubation with C1q. *J Neurosci Res* 39, no. 4: 448–56.

Wight, R. D., C. A. Tull, M. W. Deel, et al. 2012. Resveratrol effects on astrocyte function: relevance to neurodegenerative diseases. *Biochem Biophys Res Commun* 426 , no. 1: 112–15.

Williams, R. W., and K. Herrup. 1988. The control of neuron number. *Annu Rev Neurosci* 11: 423–53.

Winterbourn, C. C. 1995. Toxicity of iron and hydrogen peroxide: the Fenton reaction. *Toxicol Lett* 82–83: 969–74.

Wolozin, B., W. Kellman, P. Ruosseau, et al. 2000. Decreased prevalence of Alzheimer disease associated with 3-hydroxy-3-methyglutaryl coenzyme A reductase inhibitors. *Arch Neurol* 57, no. 10: 1439–43.

Wruck, C. J., M. E. Gotz, T. Herdegen, et al. 2008. Kavalactones protect neural cells against amyloid beta peptide-induced neurotoxicity via extracellular signal-regulated kinase 1/2-dependent nuclear factor erythroid 2-related factor 2 activation. *Mol Pharmacol* 73, no. 6: 1785–95.

Xi, Y. D., H. L. Yu, J. Ding, et al. 2012. Flavonoids protect cerebrovascular endothelial cells through Nrf2 and PI3K from beta-amyloid peptide-induced oxidative damage. *Curr Neurovasc Res* 9, no. 1: 32–41.

Xi, Y. D., H. L. Yu, W. W. Ma, et al. 2011. Genistein inhibits mitochondrial-targeted oxidative damage induced by beta-amyloid peptide 25-35 in PC12 cells. *J Bioenerg Biomembr* 43, no. 4: 399–407.

Xie, H., S. Hou, J. Jiang, et al. 2013. Rapid cell death is preceded by amyloid plaque-mediated oxidative stress. *Proc Natl Acad Sci USA* 110, no. 19: 7904–9.

Xiong, Y., X. P. Jing, X. W. Zhou, et al. 2013. Zinc induces protein phosphatase 2A inactivation and tau hyperphosphorylation through Src dependent PP2A (tyrosine 307) phosphorylation. *Neurobiol Aging* 34, no. 3: 745–56.

Yamamoto, M., T. Kiyota, M. Horiba, et al. 2007. Interferon-gamma and tumor necrosis factor-alpha regulate amyloid-beta plaque deposition and beta-secretase expression in Swedish mutant APP transgenic mice. *Am J Pathol* 170, no. 2: 680–92.

Yang, X., Y. Yang, G. Li, et al. 2008. Coenzyme Q10 attenuates beta-amyloid pathology in the aged transgenic mice with Alzheimer presenilin 1 mutation. *J Mol Neurosci* 34, no. 2: 165–71.

Yankner, B. A., and M. M. Mesulam. 1991. Seminars in medicine of the Beth Israel Hospital, Boston. Beta-Amyloid and the pathogenesis of Alzheimer's disease. *N Engl J Med* 325, no. 26: 1849–57.

Yusuf, S., G. Dagenais, J. Pogue, et al. 2000. Vitamin E supplementation and cardiovascular events in high-risk patients. The Heart Outcomes Prevention Evaluation Study Investigators. *N Eng J Med* 342, no. 3: 154–60.

Zaman, Z., S. Roche, P. Fielden, et al. 1992. Plasma concentrations of vitamins A and E and carotenoids in Alzheimer's disease. *Age Ageing* 21, no. 2: 91–94.

Zambrano, S., A. J. Blanca, M. V. Ruiz-Armenta, et al. 2013. The renoprotective effect of L-carnitine in hypertensive rats is mediated by modulation of oxidative stress-related gene expression. *Eur J Nutr* 52, no. 6: 1649–59.

Zandi, P. P., J. C. Anthony, A. S. Khachaturian, et al. 2004. Reduced risk of Alzheimer disease in users of antioxidant vitamin supplements: the Cache County Study. *Arch Neurol* 61, no. 1: 82–88.

Zara, S., M. De Colli, M. Rapino, et al. 2013. Ibuprofen and lipoic Acid conjugate neuroprotective activity is mediated by ngb/akt intracellular signaling pathway in Alzheimer's disease rat model. *Gerontology* 59, no. 3: 250–60.

Zhang, G. L., W. G. Zhang, Y. Du, et al. 2013. Edaravone ameliorates oxidative damage associated with abeta25-35 treatment in PC12 cells. *J Mol Neurosci* 50, no. 3: 494–503.

Zhang, L., G. Q. Xing, J. L. Barker, et al. 2001. Alpha-lipoic acid protects rat cortical neurons against cell death induced by amyloid and hydrogen peroxide through the Akt signalling pathway. *Neurosci Lett* 312, no. 3: 125–28.

Zhang, L. X., R. V. Cooney, and J. S. Bertram. 1992. Carotenoids up-regulate connexin43 gene expression independent of their provitamin A or antioxidant properties. *Cancer Res* 52, no. 20: 5707–12.

Zhu, J., W. Yong, X. Wu, et al. 2008. Anti-inflammatory effect of resveratrol on TNF-alpha-induced MCP-1 expression in adipocytes. *Biochem Biophys Res Commun* 369, no. 2: 471–77.

Zito, G., R. Polimanti, V. Panetta, et al. 2013. Antioxidant status and APOE genotype as susceptibility factors for neurodegeneration in Alzheimer's disease and vascular dementia. *Rejuvenation Res* 16, no. 1: 51–56.

Zou, Y., B. Hong, L. Fan, et al. 2013. Protective effect of puerarin against beta-amyloid-induced oxidative stress in neuronal cultures from rat hippocampus: involvement of the GSK-3beta/Nrf2 signaling pathway. *Free Radic Res* 47, no. 1: 55–63.

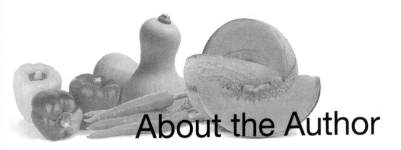

About the Author

Kedar N. Prasad, Ph.D., former president of the International Society for Nutrition and Cancer, obtained a master's degree in zoology from the University of Bihar, Ranchi, India, and his Ph.D. in radiation biology from the University of Iowa, Iowa City, in 1963. He then attended the Brookhaven National Laboratory on Long Island for postdoctoral training before joining the Department of Radiology at the University of Colorado Health Sciences Center, where he became a professor in 1980. Later he was appointed director of the Center for Vitamins and Cancer Research at the University of Colorado School of Medicine. In 1982 he was invited by the Nobel Prize Committee to nominate a candidate for the Nobel Prize in medicine, and in 1999 he was selected to deliver the Harold Harper Lecture at the meeting of the American College of Advancement in Medicine.

His published papers and articles have appeared in such illustrious publications as *Science, Nature,* and *Proceedings of the National Academy of Sciences* (PNAS). He is also the author of several book chapters and 25 books, including *Fighting Cancer with Vitamins and Antioxidants.* A member of several professional organizations, he served as an ad-hoc member of various study sections of the National Institutes of Health (NIH) and has consistently obtained NIH grants for his research.

Kedar N. Prasad is frequently an invited speaker at national and international meetings on nutrition and cancer. He began researching various types of cancers and the effects of radiation on human tissues in 1963. Over the next twenty-five years, he continued his biological research in collaboration with major universities and research labs, studying the relationships between micronutrients, cancer, and radiation, and focusing on the effects that micronutrients have on human cells and the manner in which they interact with mainstream medical therapies for many common diseases. He found that certain combinations of micronutrients, when taken in conjunction with standard treatments such as chemotherapy, enhanced and complemented the effects of these traditional therapies. The findings inspired him to further his research to determine the effects that these micronutrient combinations might have on other diseases and on general human health.

His present research interests are in the areas of radiation protection, nutrition and cancer, and nutrition and neurological diseases, particularly Alzheimer's disease and Parkinson's disease. Since 2005 he has been the chief scientific officer of the Premier Micronutrient Corporation, which produces antioxidant micronutrient formulations to promote a healthy lifestyle.

Index